Tasty Pregnancy Recipes

The Big Pregnancy Cookbook with Simple and Healthy Meal
Ideas for New Moms

By: Martha Stanford

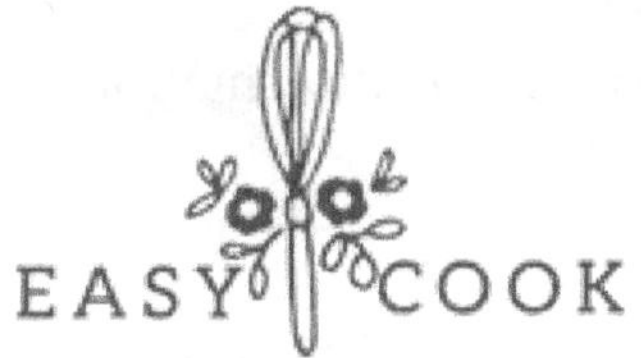

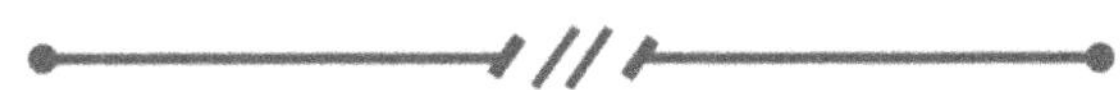

Important Notice

Dear Valued Reader,

This book is the result of my hard work and dedication. I kindly ask that you respect my intellectual property rights by not reproducing, distributing, or transmitting any part of this publication in any form or by any means without my prior written consent. This includes photocopying, recording, or using electronic or mechanical methods. However, brief quotations used in critical reviews and certain other noncommercial uses are permitted by copyright law.

I have put a great deal of effort into ensuring that the information provided in this book is both accurate and useful. However, I cannot guarantee specific results or outcomes from applying this information, as individual circumstances may vary. It is important to remember that you have the power to make your own choices and determine the path that is right for you. While I hope that the content of this book will inspire and guide you, ultimately, the way you choose to use this information is up to you.

By reading this book, you acknowledge that I shall not be held responsible for any consequences resulting from the use or misuse of the information presented.

Thank you for your understanding and for respecting the time and effort I have put into creating this work.

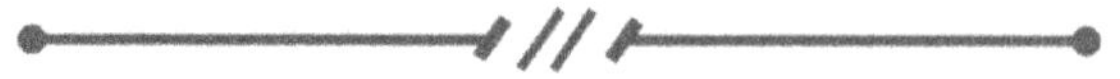

Table of Contents

Introduction

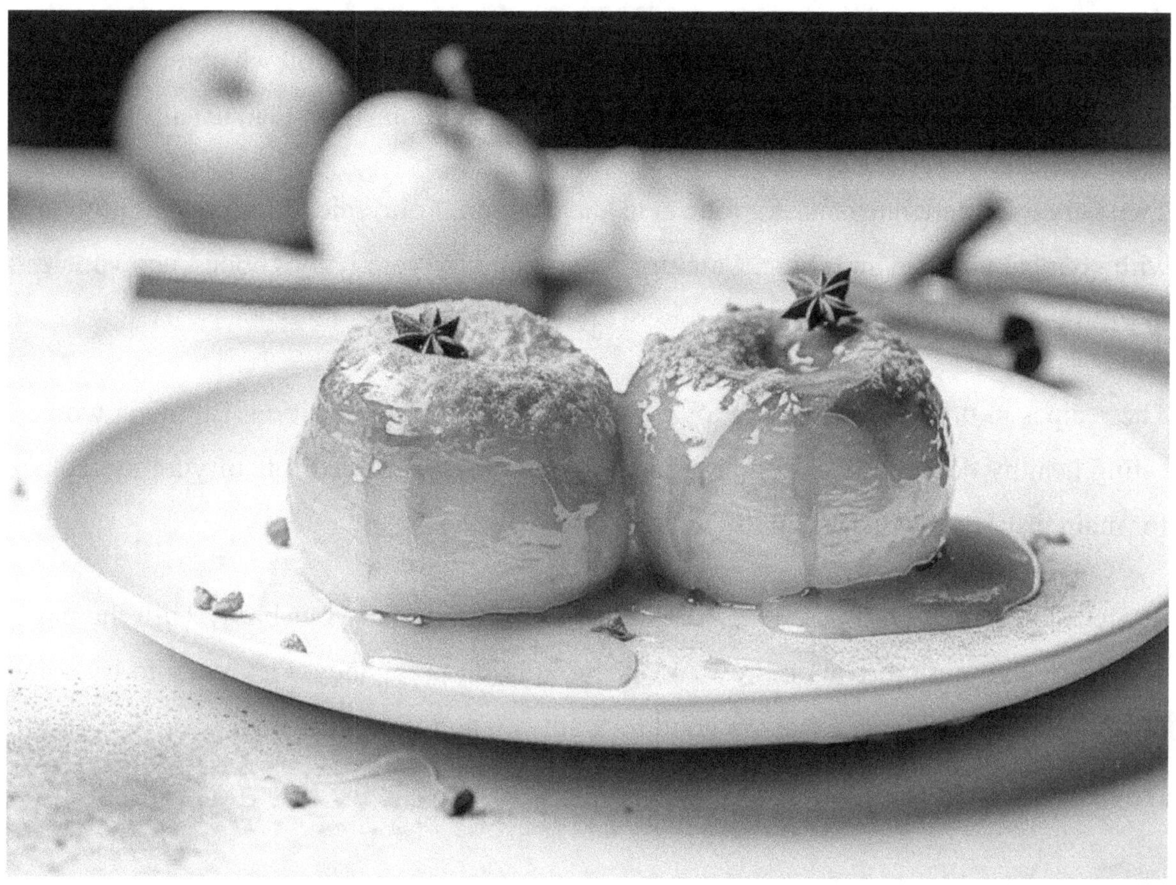

Welcome to this helpful guide for eating well during pregnancy! If you're expecting, you probably have many questions about what to eat and how much. Don't worry - this book is here to help you figure it all out.

When you're pregnant, your body needs extra calories, especially in the later months when your baby is growing fast. But it's not just about eating more - it's about eating the right foods to help your baby grow and develop.

A good pregnancy diet includes a mix of carbohydrates, proteins, vitamins, fats, and minerals. And don't forget to drink plenty of water! The US government has guidelines that can help you figure out how much of each type of food you should eat.

When you're shopping, take a look at the food labels. They'll tell you what nutrients are in the food. When you're pregnant, you need more of certain nutrients than usual.

Two very important nutrients are folic acid and calcium. Folic acid helps prevent problems with your baby's brain and spine. Calcium is important for your baby's bones, and you need to keep your own calcium levels up too.

The recipes in this book are made to give your baby the right nutrition. But don't worry - eating healthy doesn't mean giving up tasty food! We've included lots of yummy recipes for main dishes, side dishes, and snacks.

So, let's get started on this journey of eating well for you and your baby. Turn the page, and you'll find out more about how to eat right during pregnancy. Get ready to try some delicious, nutritious meals that are good for both you and your little one!

XXXXXXXXXXXXXXXXXXXXXXX

1. Lemon Shrimp Pasta

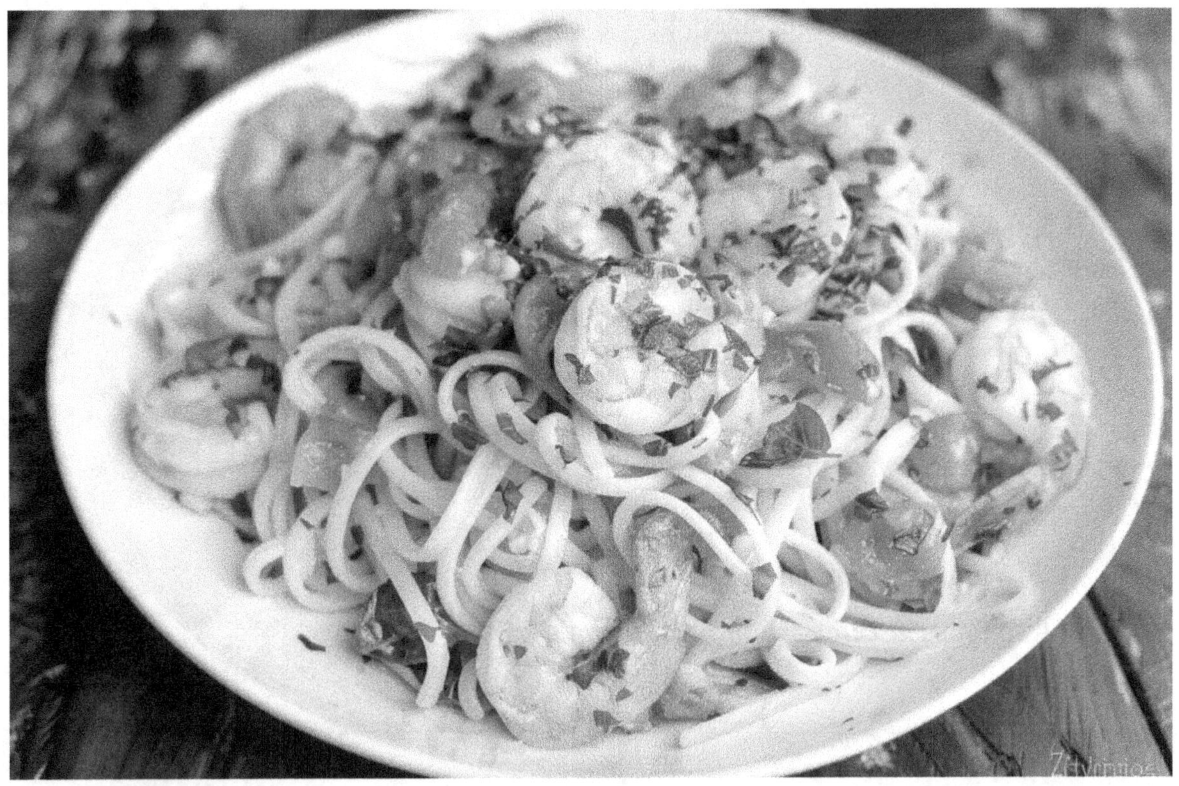

Recipe Description: This Italian-inspired dish is a hit in coastal towns. It's quick to make and tastes great. The shrimp and lemon combo gives it a fresh flavor. You'll love how the creamy sauce coats the pasta. It's perfect for a light dinner or lunch.

Preparation Time: 25 minutes

Serving size: 2 servings

Ingredients:

- 6 oz raw shrimp, peeled & deveined
- 4 oz whole-wheat fettuccine
- 1&1/2 tsp olive oil
- 1&1/2 tsp finely chopped garlic
- 1 tbsp unsalted butter
- 1/8 tsp crushed red pepper
- 2 cups loosely packed arugula
- 2 tbsp whole milk plain yogurt
- 1/2 tsp fresh lemon zest
- 1 tbsp fresh lemon juice
- 1/8 tsp kosher salt
- 3 tbsp grated Parmesan cheese + extra for garnishing
- 2 tbsp thinly sliced fresh basil (for garnish)

XXXXXXXXXXXXXXXXXXXXXXX

Instructions:

a. Boil 4 cups water in a pot. Add fettuccine, stir, and cook 7-9 minutes until just tender. Save 1/2 cup cooking water, then drain pasta.

b. Heat oil in a big non-stick pan over medium-high heat. Cook shrimp 2-3 minutes until pink and curled. Put shrimp in a bowl.

c. Melt butter in the pan over medium heat. Add garlic and red pepper. Cook for 1 minute until the garlic smells good.

d. Add arugula. Cook for 1 minute until wilted.

e. Mix in yogurt, fettuccine, and lemon zest. Add saved pasta water, 1/4 cup at a time. Toss well each time until pasta is creamy.

f. Add lemon juice, shrimp, and salt. Toss well. Turn off heat. Mix in Parmesan cheese.

g. Top with extra Parmesan and basil. Serve hot.

Special Notes:

- Try grilling the shrimp instead of pan-frying for a smoky flavor.
- For a richer sauce, swap the yogurt with mascarpone cheese. It'll make the dish creamier and more indulgent.

2. Lean Bean Joes (The Healthier Sloppy)

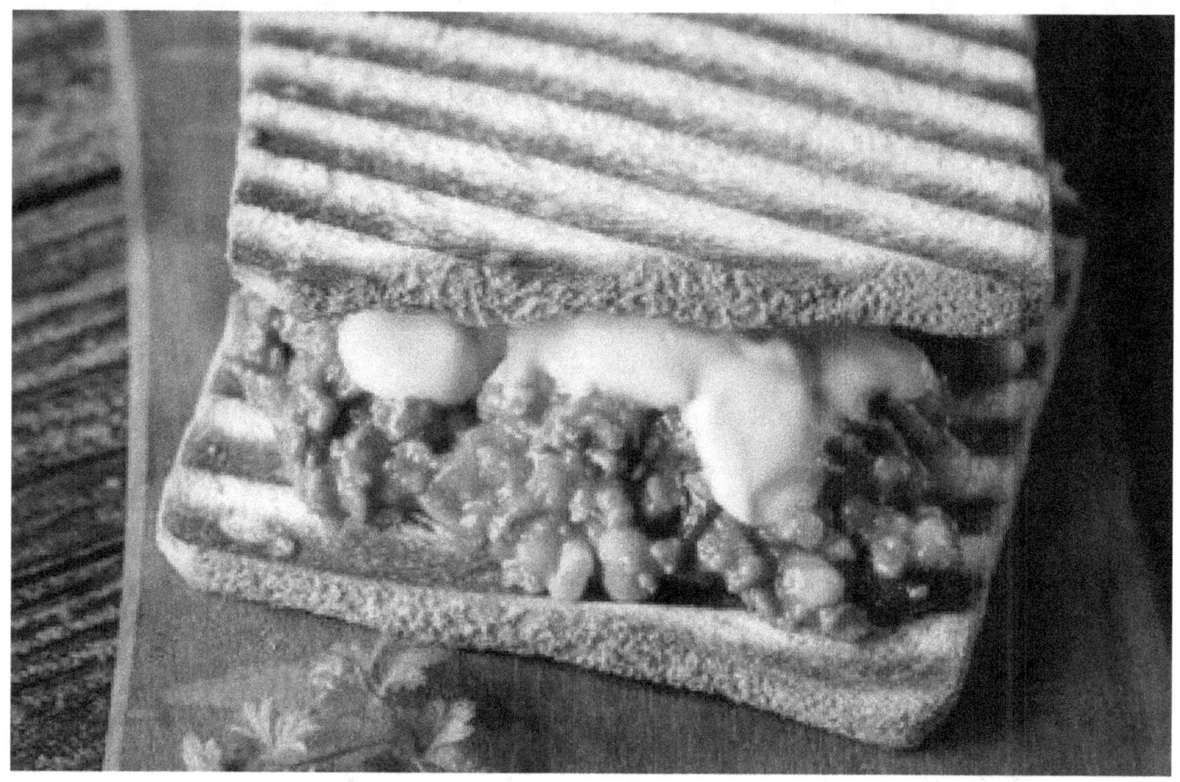

This twist on classic Sloppy Joes comes from a health-conscious cook in Ohio. It's gaining fans fast thanks to its tasty blend of beef and beans. People love it because it's filling, easy to make, and doesn't leave you feeling heavy. It's perfect for busy weeknights or casual get-togethers.

Preparation Time: 25 minutes

Serving size: 4 servings

Ingredients:

- 4 whole wheat hamburger buns, split and toasted
- 1 tablespoon olive oil
- 1 cup no-salt-added tomato sauce
- 12 oz lean ground beef (90% lean)
- 2 teaspoons chili powder
- 1 cup chopped onion
- 1 cup no-salt-added black beans, rinsed
- 1/2 teaspoon onion powder
- 1/2 teaspoon garlic powder
- 1 pinch cayenne pepper
- 3 tablespoons low-sodium ketchup
- 1 tablespoon reduced-sodium Worcestershire sauce
- 2 teaspoons spicy brown mustard
- 1 teaspoon light brown sugar

XXXXXXXXXXXXXXXXXXXXXXXX

Instructions:

a. Get a big non-stick pan hot over medium-high heat. Add the oil and beef.

b. Cook the beef for 3-4 minutes. Break it up as you go. It should be lightly brown but not fully cooked. Scoop it out with a slotted spoon into a bowl. Keep the drippings in the pan.

c. Toss the onions and beans into the pan. Cook for 4-5 minutes, stirring often. The onions should get soft.

d. Sprinkle in the garlic powder, onion powder, chili powder, and a tiny bit of cayenne. Stir for 30 seconds until it smells good.

e. Pour in the tomato sauce, ketchup, Worcestershire sauce, mustard, and brown sugar. Stir it all up. Put the beef back in.

f. Let it bubble gently. Cook for 4-5 minutes, stirring now and then. The beef should be fully cooked and the sauce a bit thicker.

g. Serve your Lean Bean Joes on the toasted whole wheat buns.

Special Notes:

- Secret flavor boost: Add a splash of apple cider vinegar to the sauce. It gives a tangy kick that makes the flavors pop.
- Veggie sneak: Grate a small zucchini and mix it in with the onions. It adds extra nutrition and keeps the meat mixture moist without changing the taste.

3. Nutty Honey Chicken Delight

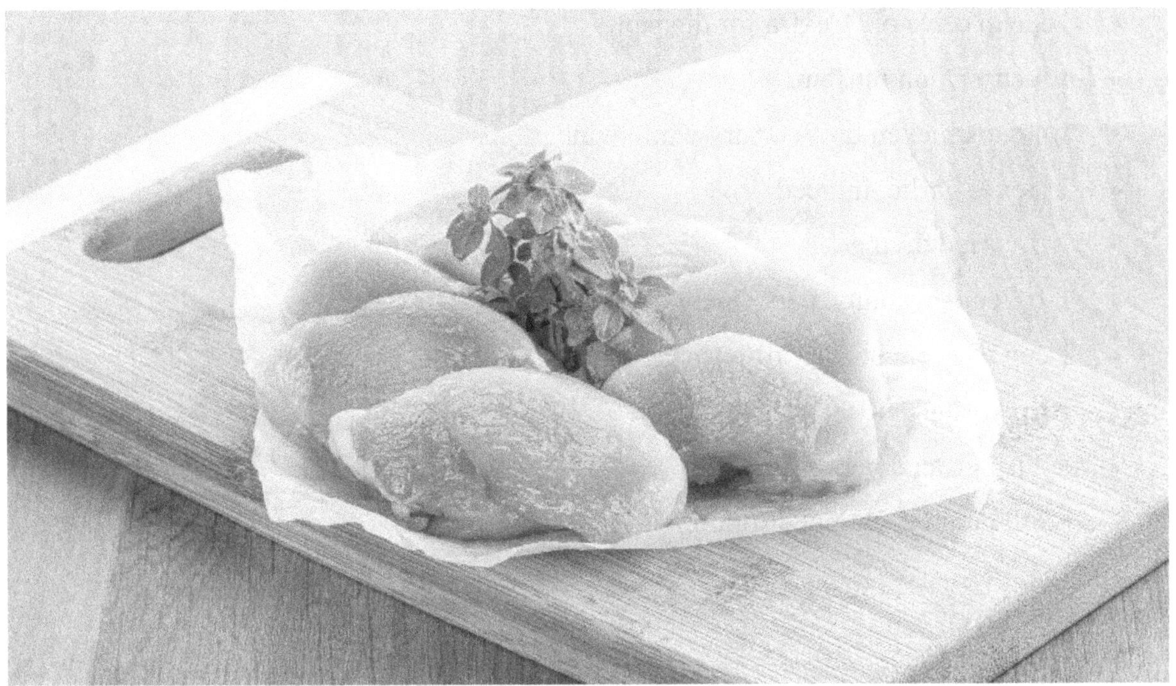

This sweet and savory chicken dish comes from a home cook in Texas. It's gotten popular at potlucks and family dinners. The chicken is coated in crunchy walnuts and drizzled with honey mustard glaze. You'll love how the flavors blend together. It's easy to make and tastes great hot or cold.

Preparation Time: 4 hours 55 minutes (including marinating)

Serving Size: 4 servings

Ingredients:

- 4 large boneless, skinless chicken breasts
- 1/3 cup olive oil + extra for the pan
- 1/4 cup Dijon mustard
- 1/4 cup chicken broth or dry white wine
- 3 cloves garlic, minced
- 1 tsp dried thyme
- 1 1/2 cups walnuts, very finely chopped
- 1 cup whole wheat or all-purpose flour
- 1 tsp kosher salt
- 1/2 tsp ground pepper
- Fresh parsley, chopped (optional, for serving)

For the honey glaze:

- 1/3 cup pure honey
- 3 tbsp Dijon mustard

xxxxxxxxxxxxxxxxxxxxxxx

Instructions:

a. Mix olive oil, wine or broth, mustard, thyme, and garlic in a zip-top bag. Add chicken, seal, and shake to coat. Chill for 4-12 hours.

b. Mix flour, walnuts, salt, and pepper in a shallow dish.

c. Take chicken out of the bag. Shake off extra marinade. Coat each piece in the walnut mix.

d. Heat oven to 425°F.

e. Heat 2 tbsp oil in an oven-safe non-stick pan over medium heat. Cook chicken for 1 minute per side.

f. Move pan to oven. Cover loosely with foil. Bake for 15-20 minutes until the chicken reaches 165°F inside.

g. Mix honey and mustard for the glaze.

h. Sprinkle parsley on chicken if you want. Serve with glaze on the side.

Special Notes:

- For extra crunch, toast the walnuts before chopping. This brings out their flavor and makes the coating even crispier.

- If you like a bit of heat, add a pinch of cayenne pepper to the walnut coating. It'll give a nice kick without overpowering the honey-mustard flavor.

4. Veggie Curry Rice Bowl (The Rainbow Delight)

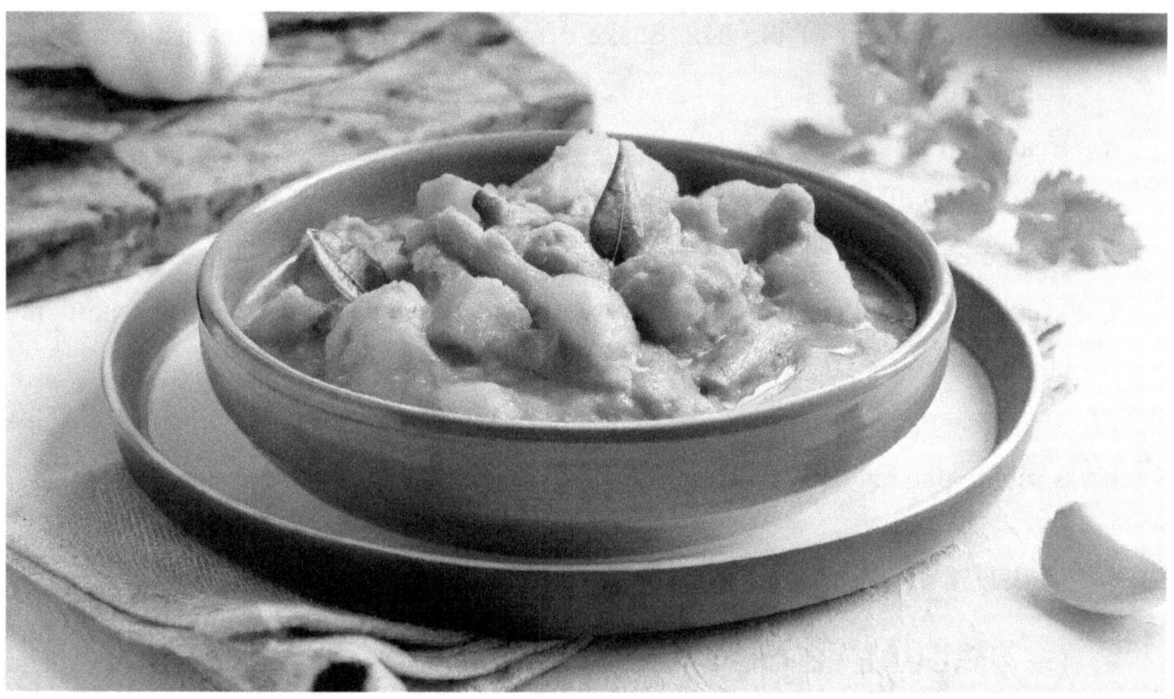

Recipe Description: This tasty dish comes from Indian-inspired cooking. It's a hit at potlucks and family dinners. The mix of veggies with curry spices makes it yummy and healthy. You'll love how the colors pop on your plate. It's easy to make and fills you up nicely.

Preparation Time: 30 minutes

Serving size: 4 servings

Ingredients:

- 1 can (7 oz) sweet corn
- 1&1/2 cups cooked rice, warmed
- 1 tablespoon vegetable oil
- 1 medium onion, peeled and sliced
- 2 teaspoons curry powder
- 2 medium carrots, peeled and diced
- 1 garlic clove, finely chopped
- 1&1/4 cups filtered water
- 1/2 small cauliflower head, florets only
- 1 large potato, peeled and cubed
- 1/3 cup low-fat natural yogurt

xxxxxxxxxxxxxxxxxxxxxxxx

Instructions:

a. Get a medium pan hot with oil. Cook the onion until it's soft and starting to brown.

b. Toss in the garlic and curry powder. Let it cook for about a minute to wake up the flavors.

c. Pour in the water. Add your veggies: carrots, potatoes, cauliflower, and corn.

d. Let it bubble up, then turn down the heat. Put a lid on and let it simmer for 13-15 minutes.

e. Take the pan off the heat. Stir in the yogurt. Put it back on low heat.

f. Give it 2 more minutes of gentle cooking. Scoop it over your warm rice and enjoy!

Special Notes:

- Secret flavor boost: Try adding a pinch of garam masala at the end for an extra kick of Indian flavor.
- Veggie swap trick: Feel free to switch up the veggies based on what's in your fridge. Bell peppers or green peas work great too!

5. Singapore Noodle Stir-Fry

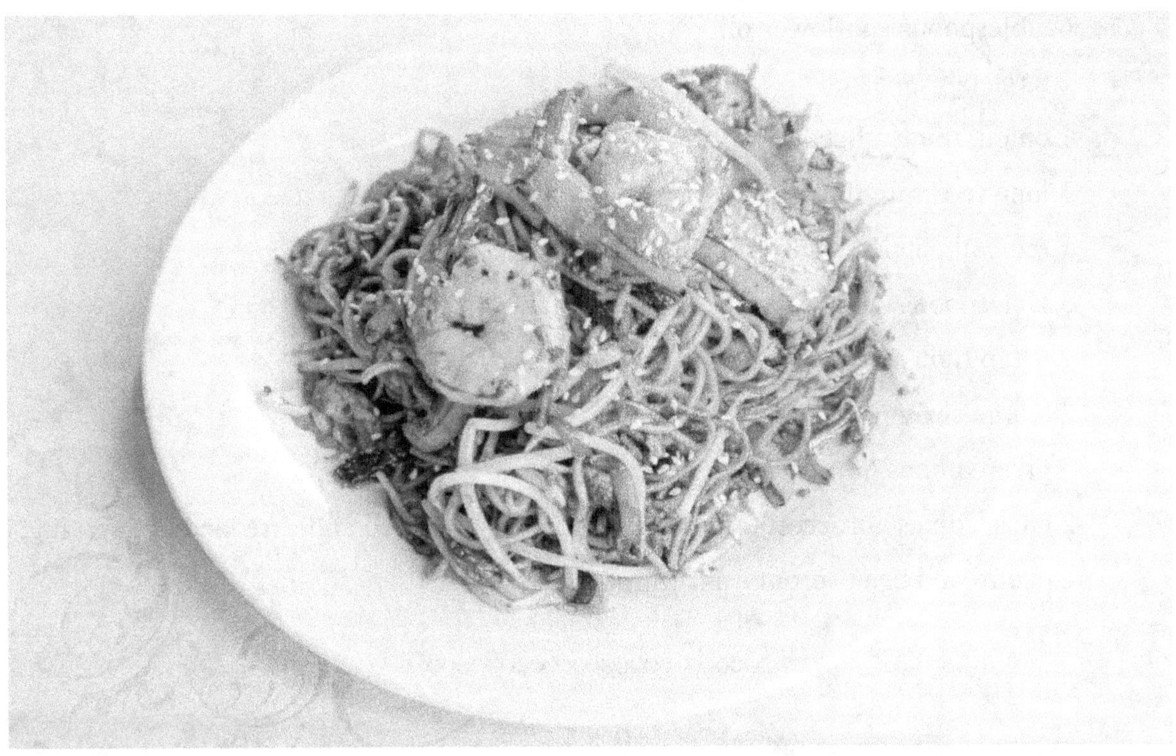

This tasty noodle dish isn't from Singapore at all - it's actually a Cantonese creation! It's super popular in Chinese restaurants worldwide. With curry-flavored noodles, veggies, and shrimp, it's a quick and filling meal. Perfect for chilly nights when you want something warm and satisfying.

Preparation Time: 35 minutes

Serving size: 4 servings

Ingredients:

- 1-pound thin egg noodles, cooked according to package instructions
- 6 tablespoons sunflower oil
- 2 large eggs, beaten
- 1 onion, thinly sliced
- 1 long red chili, thinly sliced
- 1 red bell pepper, thinly sliced
- 5 tablespoons curry powder
- 1/4 cup light soy sauce
- 24 large shrimp, peeled with tails on
- 3 green onions, thinly sliced
- 2 cups Chinese broccoli (or regular broccoli), blanched and shredded For serving:
- Cilantro and bean sprouts, as desired

xxxxxxxxxxxxxxxxxxxxxxx

Instructions:

a. Heat 1 tablespoon of oil in a wok over medium-high heat. Pour in beaten eggs and swirl to cook. Remove and slice the egg.

b. Add 2 tablespoons oil to the wok and crank up the heat. Toss in onions and chili. Cook until onions turn golden, about 1-2 minutes. Add bell pepper and cook for 2-3 minutes until soft. Take the veggies out of the wok.

c. Throw in the curry powder and cook for a minute or two. Add the cooked noodles and soy sauce. Toss well to coat the noodles, then remove from the wok.

d. Heat the remaining oil in the wok. Cook the shrimp for 2 minutes per side until they turn pink and slightly crispy.

e. Toss in broccoli and green onions. Cook for a minute. Add the noodles and cooked veggies back to the wok. Mix everything together.

f. Sprinkle with bean sprouts and cilantro if you like. Serve hot and enjoy!

Special Notes:

- Secret flavor boost: Add a splash of fish sauce along with the soy sauce for extra umami goodness.
- Veggie swap: Feel free to use whatever veggies you have on hand - carrots, snow peas, or baby corn work great too!

6. Cucumber Yogurt Salad: The Cool Crunch

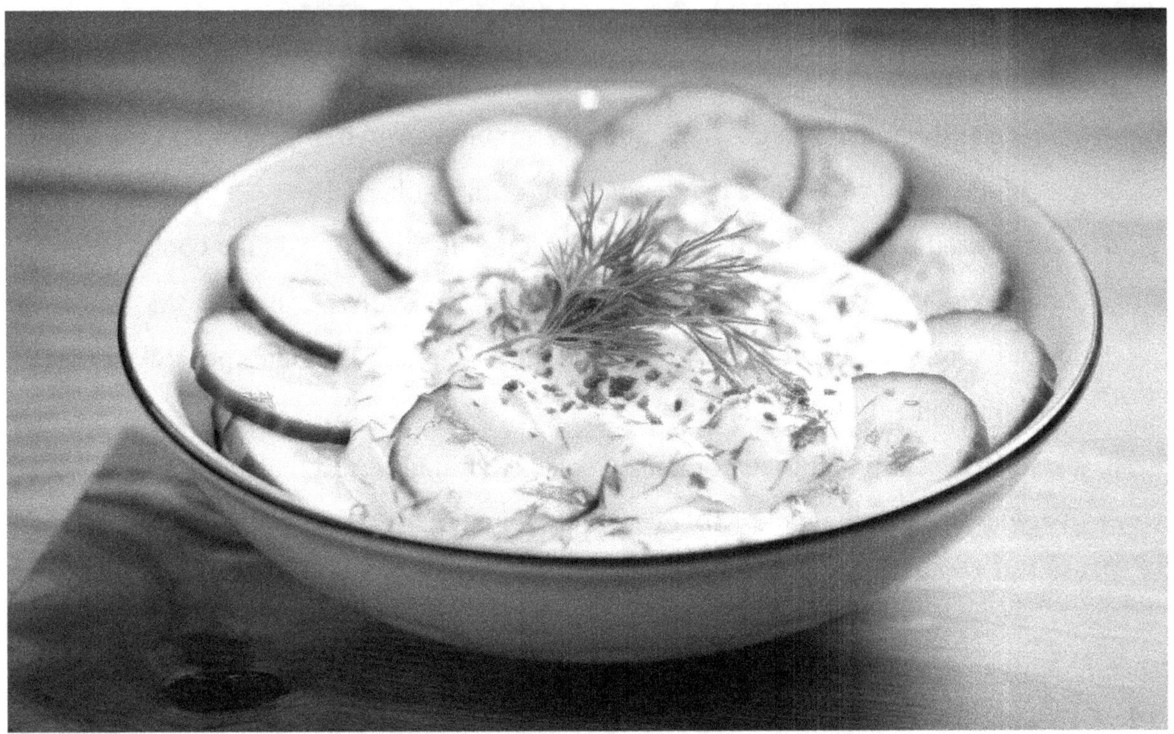

Recipe Description: This easy salad comes from the Middle East. It's popular in hot weather and goes great with spicy food. The main ingredients are cucumber and yogurt. You'll love how refreshing it is. It's also good for babies because it has lots of good stuff in it.

Preparation Time: 10 minutes

Serving size: 4 servings

Ingredients:

- 2 cucumbers, peeled, quartered lengthwise, and sliced
- 1 cup low-fat plain yogurt
- 1 tsp dried dill
- Kosher salt and ground pepper to taste

XXXXXXXXXXXXXXXXXXXXXXXX

Instructions:

a. Check if the cucumbers taste bitter. If they do, put them in slightly salty water for about 30 minutes. Then rinse and dry them.
b. Mix all the ingredients in a bowl. Don't stir too hard.
c. Add salt and pepper how you like it.
d. Serve and enjoy!

Special Notes:

- For extra crunch, leave some cucumber skin on when peeling.
- Try adding a small, finely chopped onion for a flavor kick. Red onion works great and adds a nice color too.

7. Liver & Onions Delight

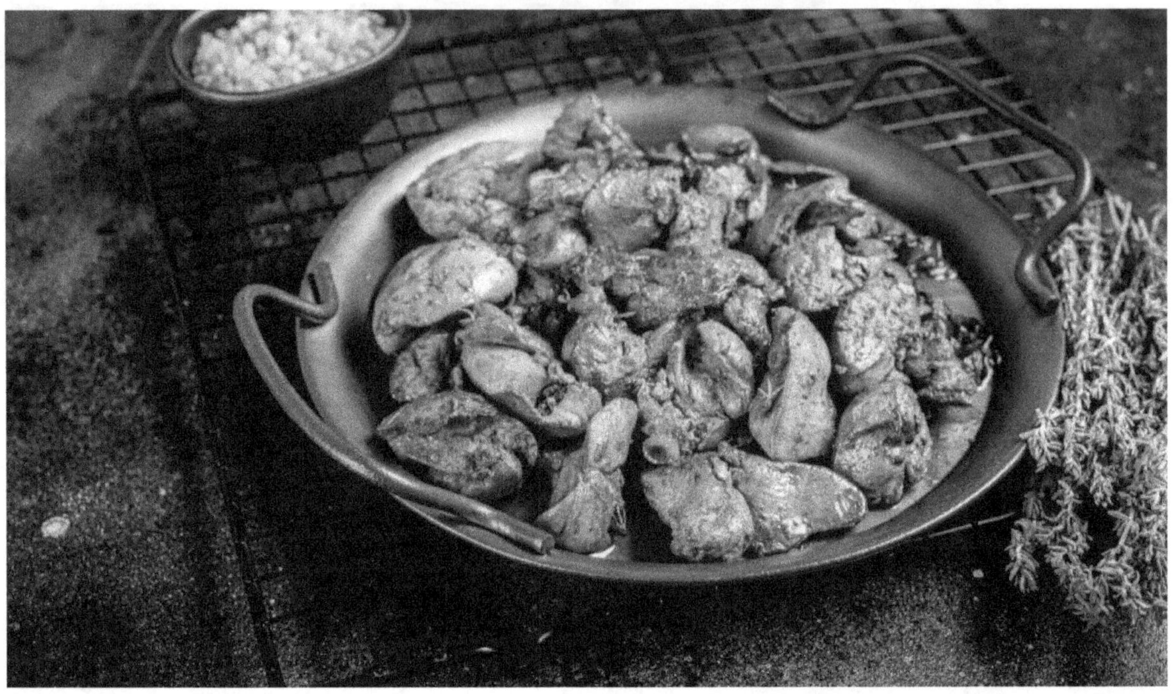

This liver and onions recipe turns a classic dish into a family favorite. Born in American kitchens, it's a go-to for meat lovers. With tender beef liver and sweet onions as stars, it's a tasty way to get your iron. Even if you're not a liver fan, give this a try - you might be surprised!

Preparation Time: 50 minutes

Serving size: 4 servings

Ingredients:

- 2 lbs. beef liver, sliced
- 1&1/2 cups low-fat milk, plus extra if needed
- 1/4 cup unsalted butter
- 2 large onions, sliced into rings
- 1 cup all-purpose flour, plus extra if needed
- Kosher salt and ground pepper to taste

XXXXXXXXXXXXXXXXXXXXXXXX

Instructions:

a. Clean the liver slices under cold water. Put them in a bowl.

b. Pour in enough milk to cover the liver. Let it sit while you cook the onions, or soak for an hour if you have time.

c. In a big pan, melt 2 tablespoons of butter over medium heat. Cook the onion rings until soft. Take them out and set aside.

d. Melt the rest of the butter in the same pan. Mix salt and pepper into the flour in a shallow dish.

e. Take the liver out of the milk and pat dry. Coat each slice in the seasoned flour.

f. Turn up the heat to medium-high. Once the butter is hot, add the floured liver slices.

g. Cook until the bottom is brown, then flip. Brown the other side too.

h. Put the onions back in the pan. Lower the heat to medium and cook a bit longer if you like.

i. Serve hot and enjoy your liver and onions!

Special Notes:

- For extra tenderness, soak the liver in buttermilk instead of regular milk. The acidity helps soften the meat.
- Try adding a splash of balsamic vinegar when cooking the onions. It gives a nice sweet and tangy kick that goes great with liver.

8. Chickpea & Greens Turkey Stew

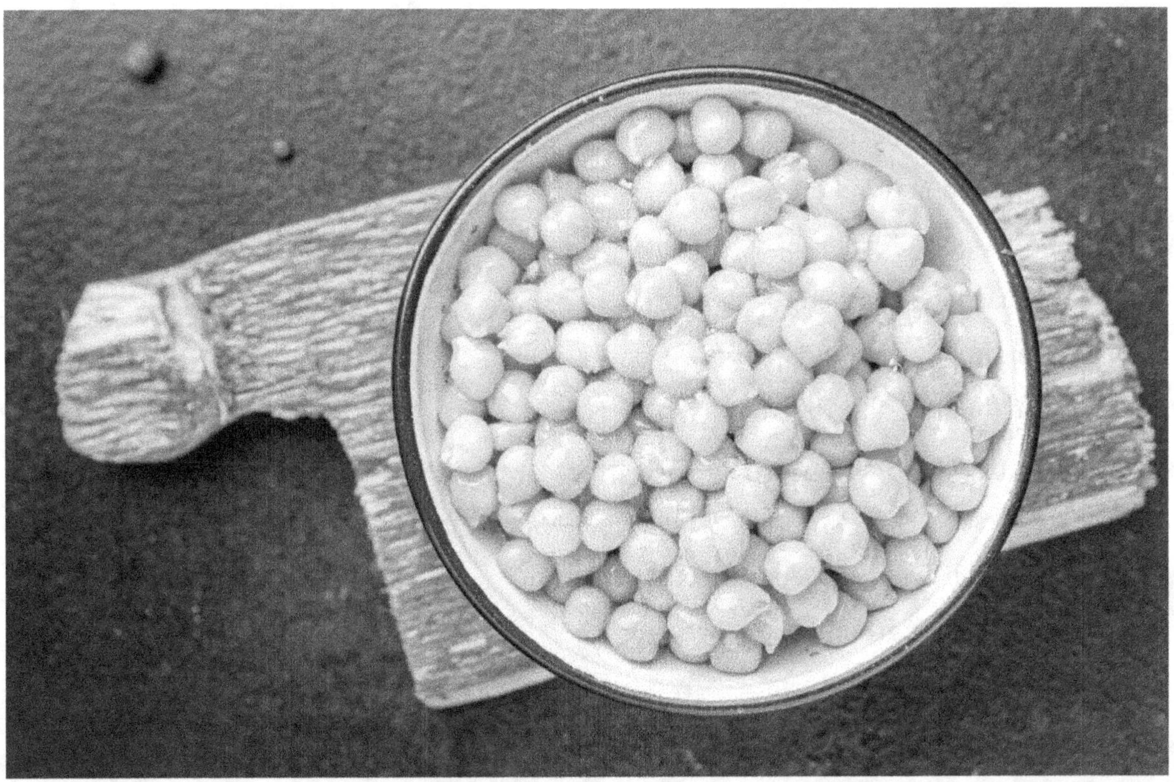

This hearty stew comes from an old Italian family recipe. It's popular among health-conscious eaters and busy parents. With chickpeas, turkey, and spinach as the stars, it's a tasty way to pack in protein and veggies. You'll love how it warms you up on chilly days.

Preparation Time: 35 minutes

Serving size: 4 servings

Ingredients:

- 2 cans (15 oz each) low-sodium chickpeas, rinsed
- 8 oz individually quick-frozen spinach
- 1 tablespoon olive oil
- 12 oz ground lean turkey
- 1/2 teaspoon dried oregano
- 1/2 teaspoon fennel seeds, crushed
- 1/2 teaspoon crushed red pepper
- 1 medium onion, chopped
- 2 medium carrots, diced
- 4 garlic cloves, minced
- 3 tablespoons no-salt-added tomato paste
- 1 carton (32 oz) low-sodium chicken broth
- 1/4 teaspoon ground pepper
- 1/8 teaspoon kosher salt
- 1/4 cup grated Parmesan cheese (optional, for garnish)

XXXXXXXXXXXXXXXXXXXXXXXX

Instructions:

a. Grab one can of chickpeas and mash them up with a fork or potato masher. Set aside.

b. Get a big pot hot over medium-high heat and add the oil. Throw in the turkey, oregano, fennel seeds, and red pepper. Break up the turkey as it cooks for about 2-3 minutes until it's no longer pink.

c. Toss in the onions, carrots, and garlic. Keep stirring and cooking for 3-4 minutes until they smell good and soften up. Add the tomato paste and cook for another 30 seconds, stirring the whole time.

d. Now add both the whole and mashed chickpeas, broth, salt, and pepper to the pot. Cover it up and let it come to a simmer. Turn the heat down to medium, keep it covered, and let it bubble away for 9-10 minutes. This lets all the flavors mix and the veggies get tender.

e. Time for the spinach! Turn the heat back up to medium-high. Add the spinach and stir it in for 1-2 minutes until it's heated through.

f. Scoop the stew into bowls. If you want, sprinkle a tablespoon of Parmesan cheese on top before serving.

Special Notes:

- Secret flavor boost: Try adding a splash of lemon juice right before serving. It brightens up the whole dish!
- Texture trick: For a thicker stew, use an immersion blender to partially blend some of the chickpeas and veggies right in the pot. This creates a creamier base without adding any extra ingredients.

9. One-Pan Wonder: The Lazy Lasagna

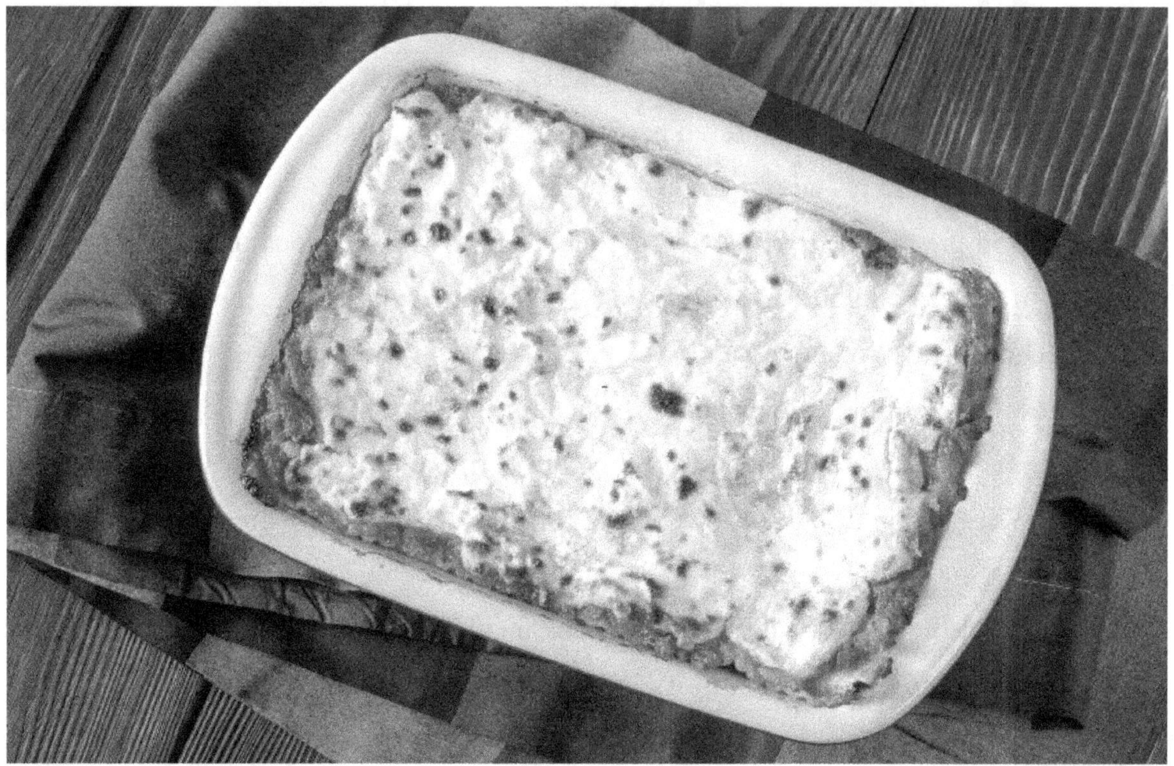

This quick lasagna hack was born in busy kitchens across America. It's a favorite for those who love Italian flavors but don't have time for layering. With ground beef, ravioli, and gooey cheese, it's a crowd-pleaser that comes together in no time. You'll love how easy and tasty it is!

Preparation Time: 25 minutes

Serving size: 6 servings

Ingredients:

- 24 oz package refrigerated or frozen cheese ravioli
- 8 oz fresh small mozzarella balls
- 1 lb. lean ground beef
- 1/2 tsp garlic powder
- 1&1/2 tsp dried oregano
- 1/2 tsp kosher salt
- 1/4 tsp ground pepper
- 28 oz can crushed tomatoes (no salt added)
- 1/4 cup fresh basil, chopped

XXXXXXXXXXXXXXXXXXXXXXXX

Instructions:

a. Turn on your oven's broiler. Get a big pot of water boiling.

b. Cook the ravioli as the package says. Drain and set aside.

c. In a large, oven-safe skillet, cook the beef over medium-high heat. Break it up as it cooks, about 4-5 minutes until it's no longer pink.

d. Add the garlic powder, oregano, salt, and pepper to the beef. Stir well.

e. Pour in the tomatoes and add the basil. Let it bubble gently.

f. Mix in the cooked ravioli and half of the mozzarella balls.

g. Sprinkle the rest of the mozzarella on top.

h. Carefully put the skillet in the oven. Broil for 2-3 minutes until the cheese melts and gets bubbly.

i. Take it out and serve hot.

Special Notes:

- For a fun twist, try using flavored ravioli like spinach or mushroom instead of plain cheese.
- If you like it spicy, add a pinch of red pepper flakes to the beef while cooking. It'll give your lazy lasagna a nice kick!

10. Prosciutto Picnic Plate

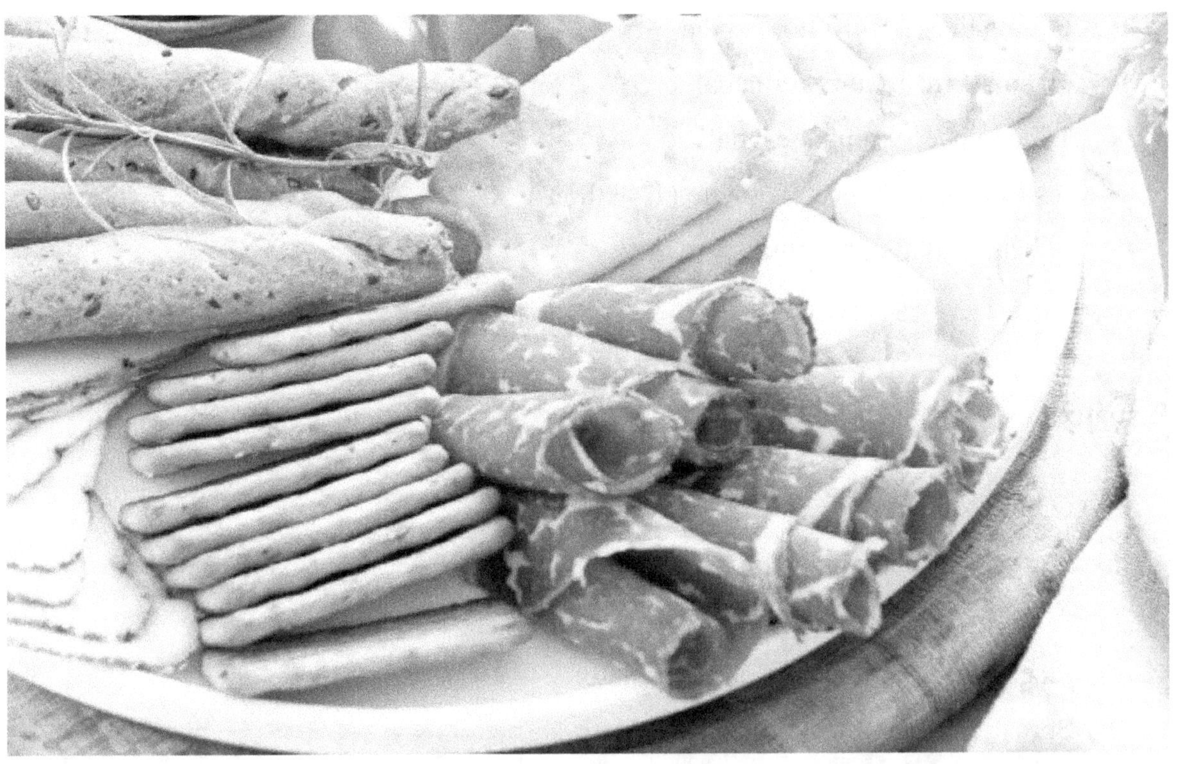

This Italian-inspired dish is a hit at summer gatherings. It's easy to make and tastes great. The mix of salty prosciutto, sweet melon, and creamy mozzarella is perfect for a light meal. People love it because it's simple but looks fancy.

Preparation Time: 10 minutes

Serving size: 2

Ingredients:

- 1 cup cantaloupe, cubed
- 6 thin slices prosciutto, halved
- 10 small fresh mozzarella balls
- 1/2 cup cherry tomatoes, halved
- 6 slices whole-wheat baguette (1/4" thick)
- 1/2 cup unsalted hazelnuts

XXXXXXXXXXXXXXXXXXXXXXXX

Instructions:

a. Grab two plates.

b. Put half the cantaloupe on each plate.

c. Add 3 halved prosciutto slices to each plate.

d. Place 5 mozzarella balls on each plate.

e. Spread half the tomatoes on each plate.

f. Add 3 baguette slices to each plate.

g. Sprinkle 1/4 cup hazelnuts on each plate.

h. Serve and enjoy your fancy picnic plate!

Special Notes:

- Try drizzling a bit of honey over the cantaloupe for extra sweetness.
- Toast the hazelnuts in a dry pan for 2-3 minutes to bring out their flavor.

11. Spicy Chicken Fajita Pasta

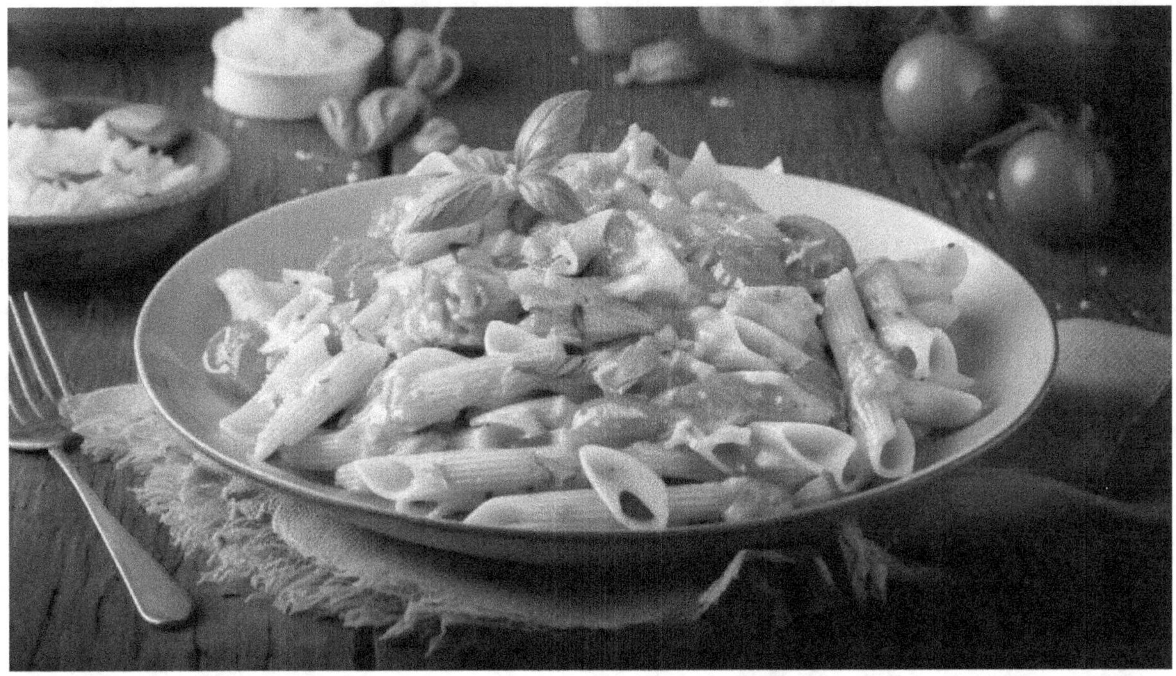

This Mexican American fusion dish blends fajita flavors with pasta. Born in Tex-Mex kitchens, it's a hit at potlucks and family dinners. Juicy chicken, colorful peppers, and penne come together in a spicy dance. You'll love how the zesty seasoning coats every bite.

Preparation Time: 45 minutes

Serving size: 4 servings

Ingredients:

- 1-pound boneless, skinless chicken thighs, trimmed and sliced
- 1/4 cup olive oil
- 2 teaspoons ground cumin
- 1 tablespoon chili powder
- 1/2 teaspoon ground chipotle
- 3/4 teaspoon kosher salt
- 1 medium red bell pepper, halved crosswise and thinly sliced
- 1 medium yellow bell pepper, halved crosswise and thinly sliced
- 1 medium onion, halved and sliced
- 8 ounces whole wheat penne
- 2 tablespoons fresh lime juice
- 1/4 cup fresh cilantro, chopped
- Sour cream or Pico de Gallo for serving (optional)

XXXXXXXXXXXXXXXXXXXXXXX

Instructions:

a. Heat your oven to 400°F. Grab a big baking sheet and spray it with cooking spray.

b. Mix 2 tablespoons olive oil, cumin, chili powder, chipotle, and 1/2 teaspoon salt in a big bowl. Toss in the chicken strips, peppers, and onions. Stir until everything is coated.

c. Spread this mix on your baking sheet in one layer. Roast for about 15 minutes.

d. Switch the oven to broil. Cook for 5 more minutes until the veggies get some char and the chicken's done.

e. While that's cooking, boil some water and cook your penne. Follow the box instructions.

f. In a big pot, mix the last of the olive oil, salt, and the lime juice. Add your pasta and the chicken mix. Toss it all together.

g. Sprinkle cilantro over the top and give it one last stir.

h. Serve it up! Add some sour cream or Pico de Gallo if you want.

Special Notes:

- Prep hack: Freeze lime juice in ice cube trays. Pop one out for an instant flavor boost!

- Secret ingredient: Try adding a splash of tequila to the chicken marinade for an extra kick of flavor. Just a tablespoon will do the trick!

12. Beef Skewer Delight: Teriyaki Twist

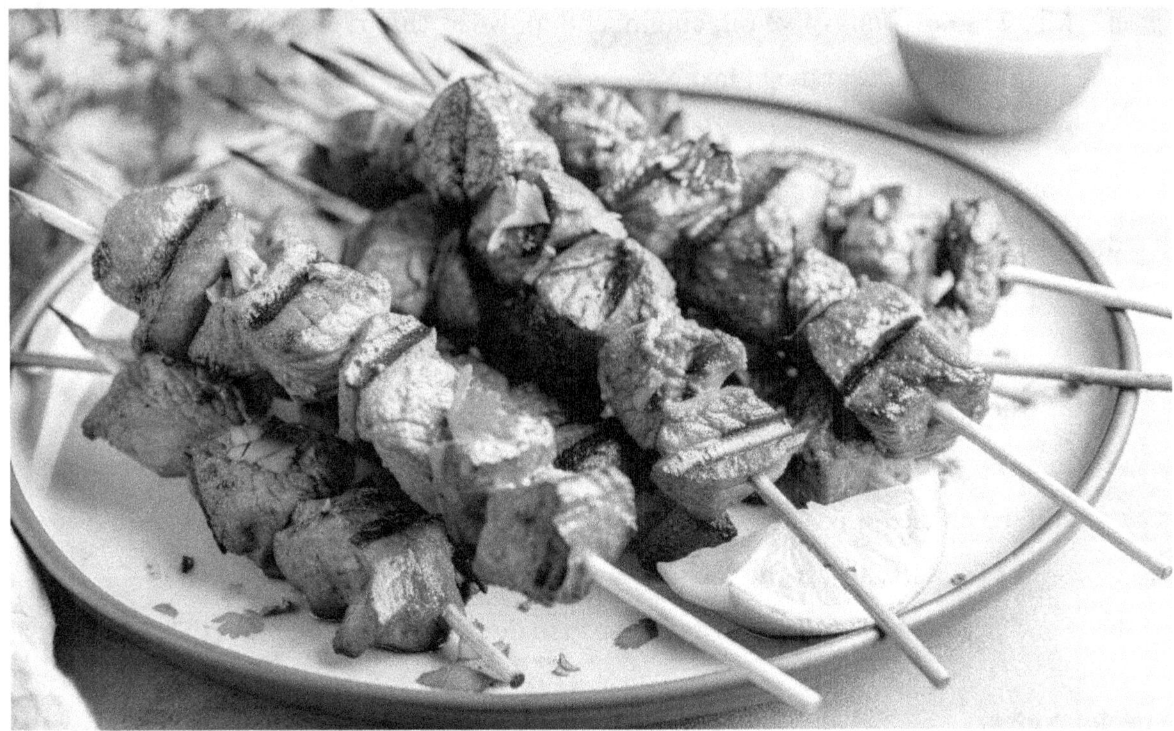

This Japanese-inspired dish puts a tasty spin on beef skewers. It's a hit at barbecues and family dinners. The tender beef soaks up the teriyaki flavor, and the fresh salad adds a nice crunch. It's quick to make and sure to become a favorite in your home.

Preparation Time: 30 minutes

Serving Size: 4 servings

Ingredients:

- 9 oz snow peas, halved lengthwise
- 1&1/2 pounds thinly sliced beef steak
- 1/3 cup low sodium teriyaki sauce
- 1 Lebanese cucumber, thinly sliced
- 2 oz baby mixed salad leaves
- 2 cups jasmine rice

For the dressing:

- 1 tsp sesame oil
- 1 tbsp rice vinegar
- 1 tbsp Japanese sweet rice wine
- 1 tbsp light soy sauce
- 1-2 tsp wasabi paste (adjust to taste)
- 1 tsp granulated sugar

XXXXXXXXXXXXXXXXXXXXXXXX

Instructions:

a.   Soak bamboo skewers in water. If using metal skewers, skip this step.

b.   Fold beef slices in half and thread onto skewers. Place in a shallow dish.

c.   Pour teriyaki sauce over the beef. Let it sit for 5-7 minutes.

d.   Boil water in a pan with a pinch of salt. Cook snow peas for 1 minute until tender. Drain and rinse with cold water.

e.   Mix snow peas, cucumber, and salad leaves in a bowl.

f.   Make the dressing: Whisk all dressing ingredients in a small bowl. Pour over the salad and toss.

g.   Heat a pan over medium-high. Cook skewers for 2 minutes per side until done and slightly charred.

h.   Cook rice according to package instructions.

i.   Serve beef skewers with rice and salad on the side.

Special Notes:

- For extra flavor, grate some fresh ginger into the teriyaki sauce before marinating the beef.
- If you're not a fan of wasabi, try adding a squeeze of lime juice to the dressing instead. It'll give a nice tang that complements the teriyaki beef.

13. Spicy Salmon Tacos: The Fish Fiesta

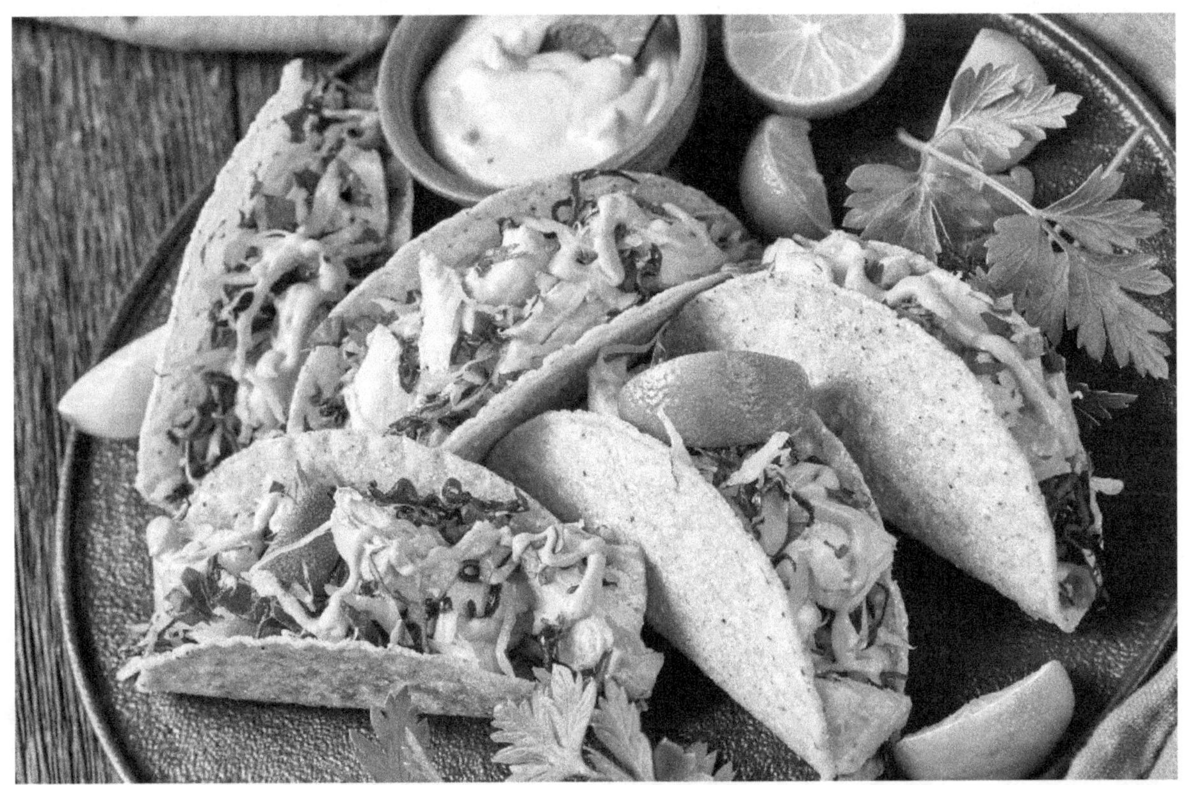

These tacos are a hit in California. They mix salmon with Mexican flavors. People love them because they're tasty and healthy. The main stars are fresh salmon, avocado, and a zesty chipotle kick. You'll want to make them again and again.

Preparation Time: 20 minutes

Cooking Time: 20 minutes

Serving Size: 8 servings

Ingredients:

- 1-pound wild Alaskan salmon fillet, cut into 4 pieces
- 4 teaspoons olive oil
- 2 tablespoons light mayonnaise
- 1 teaspoon fresh lime juice
- 2 teaspoons chipotle chili powder
- 2 teaspoons finely grated fresh orange zest
- 2 teaspoons granulated sugar
- 8 (6-inch) corn tortillas
- Sea salt, to taste
- 1 avocado, mashed
- Cucumber-apple salsa, as needed
- 1 cup finely shredded cabbage

xxxxxxxxxxxxxxxxxxxxxxxx

Instructions:

a. Turn on your oven to 350°F.

b. Mix mayo and lime juice in a small bowl.

c. In another bowl, mix chipotle powder, sugar, and orange zest. Coat salmon with 1 teaspoon oil, then rub with the spice mix. Let it sit for 5 minutes.

d. Wrap tortillas in foil and warm in the oven for 7-9 minutes.

e. Heat a grill pan. Add salt to the salmon. Cook on high for 2-3 minutes per side until brown and cooked through.

f. Break salmon into chunks. Put avocado on warm tortillas. Add salmon, salsa, and cabbage. Drizzle with the lime mayo. Serve right away.

Special Notes:

- For extra zing, pickle the cabbage in lime juice and a pinch of salt for 30 minutes before using.
- Try grilling pineapple chunks and adding them to the tacos for a sweet and tangy twist.

14. Chicken Cobb Bowl

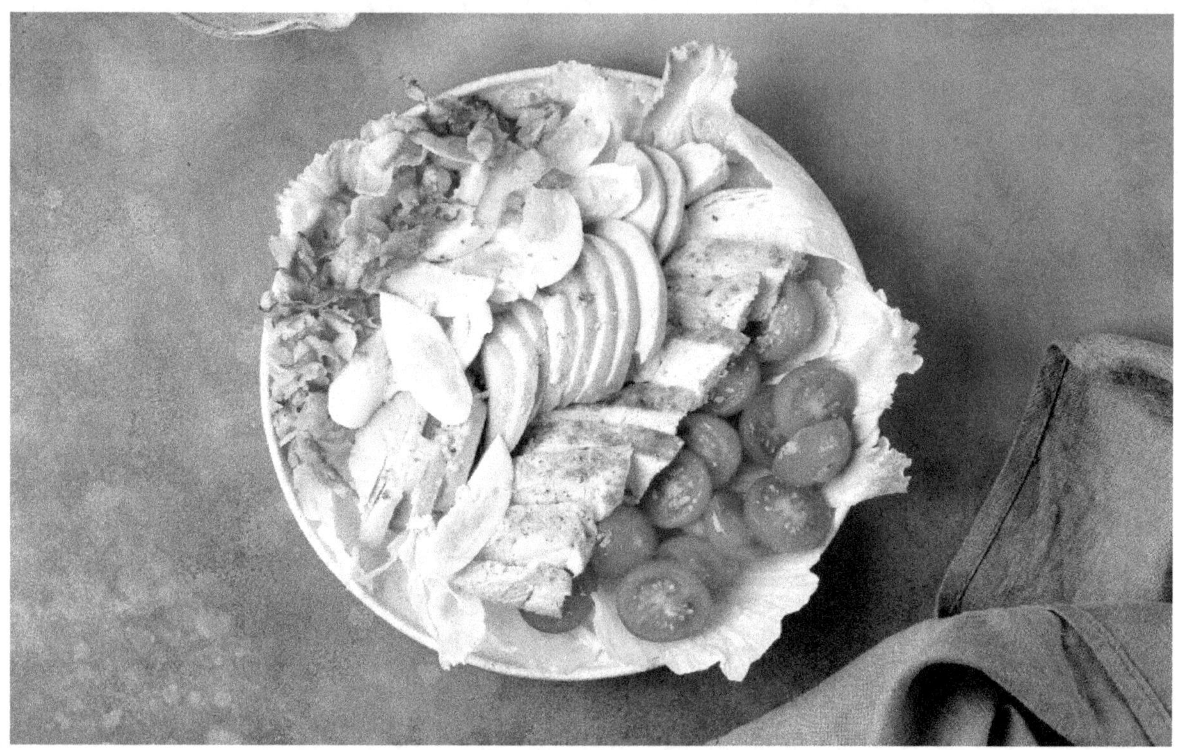

This quick and easy salad is a great way to use up leftover chicken. It's packed with veggies, protein, and flavor. Popular with American diners, the Cobb salad is a filling meal that won't leave you hungry. You'll love how fast it comes together and how good it tastes.

Preparation Time: 10 minutes

Serving size: 1 serving

Ingredients:

- 2 cups chopped romaine lettuce
- 2 tablespoons bottled blue cheese salad dressing
- 1/4 cup chopped tomato
- 1/4 cup chopped cucumber
- 1/4 cup sliced button mushrooms
- 3 oz cubed or strip-cut roasted or grilled chicken breast
- 1/2 hard-boiled egg, chopped
- 1/4 cup no-salt-added cannellini beans, drained and rinsed

XXXXXXXXXXXXXXXXXXXXXXXX

Instructions:

a. Grab a medium bowl and toss in the lettuce.
b. Pour 1 tablespoon of the dressing over the lettuce and mix it up well.
c. Now for the fun part - make rows of your toppings on the lettuce. Put the tomatoes, mushrooms, cucumbers, chicken, beans, and eggs in separate lines.
d. Finish it off by drizzling the last tablespoon of dressing on top.
e. Your Lazy Leftover Legend is ready to eat!

Special Notes:

- Try adding some crumbled bacon or avocado for extra richness. They're not in the original recipe, but they're classic Cobb salad ingredients that can take this dish to the next level.
- If you're out of blue cheese dressing, don't sweat it. Ranch or a simple olive oil and vinegar mix works great too. Just use what you have in the fridge!

15. Korean Beef Balls with Noodles

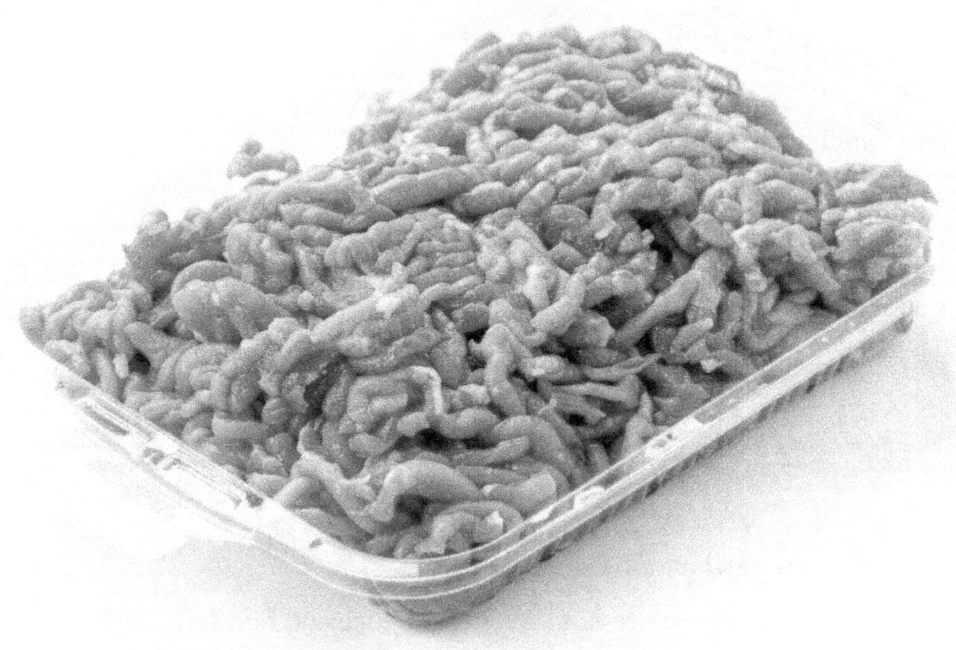

This Korean-inspired dish is a hit in many homes. It mixes juicy meatballs with chewy udon noodles and fresh veggies. The sauce is tangy and sweet. It's quick to make but tastes like you spent hours in the kitchen. You'll love how the flavors come together in each bite.

Preparation Time: 1 hour 30 minutes

Serving size: 4 servings

Ingredients:

For the meatballs:

- 1 lb. ground beef
- 1 tbsp oyster sauce
- 1 tbsp tomato sauce
- 1 tbsp olive oil

For the noodles and veggies:

- 5 oz dried udon noodles
- 7 oz broad beans, blanched and peeled
- 1 2/3 cups frozen peas, blanched

For the dressing:

- 1 cup low-sodium chicken stock
- 1/4 cup light soy sauce
- 1 tbsp rice wine vinegar
- 1 tsp sesame oil
- 1 tsp brown sugar
- 1 tbsp white sesame seeds, toasted
- Juice of 1 fresh lime
- 2 tsp mild mustard

For serving:

- Coriander
- Kimchi

Instructions:

a. Mix beef with oyster and tomato sauces in a big bowl.

b. Shape into 20 small, flat meatballs. Chill for 30 minutes.

c. Cook meatballs in olive oil over medium-low heat for 6-7 minutes, turning often. Set aside.

d. For the dressing, mix all ingredients in a pan. Heat until it simmers, then keep warm.

e. Cook udon noodles as per package instructions. Drain.

f. Add noodles, peas, and beans to the warm dressing. Mix well.

g. Put noodle mix in bowls. Top with meatballs, coriander, and kimchi.

h. Serve and enjoy your Seoul Bowl Surprise!

Special Notes:

- For extra flavor, add a splash of gochujang (Korean chili paste) to the meatball mix.
- Try swapping half the beef for ground pork to make the meatballs even juicier.

16. Crustless Mushroom Spinach Pie (The Veggie Wheel)

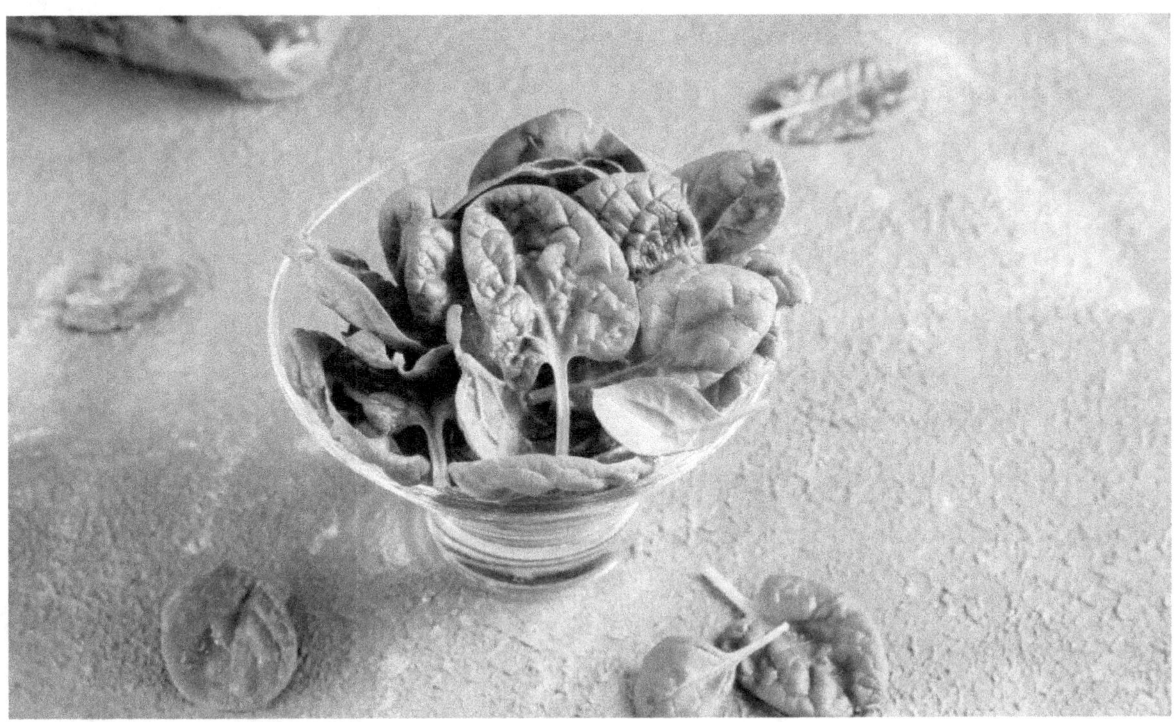

This easy-to-make vegetarian dish comes from France. It's a hit at brunches and potlucks. The stars are mushrooms, spinach, and Gruyere cheese. You'll love how the flavors blend together. It's like a quiche without the fussy crust, making it simpler to prepare.

Preparation Time: 25 minutes

Cooking Time: 30 minutes

Serving Size: 6 servings

Ingredients:

- 5 oz fresh baby spinach, coarsely chopped
- 2 tablespoons olive oil
- 8 oz mixed fresh mushrooms (button, shiitake, or cremini), sliced
- 1&1/2 cups sweet onion, thinly sliced
- 1 tablespoon garlic, thinly sliced
- 6 large eggs
- 1/4 cup whole milk
- 1/4 cup half & half
- 1 tablespoon Dijon mustard
- 1 tablespoon fresh thyme leaves + extra for garnish
- 1/4 teaspoon kosher salt
- 1/4 teaspoon ground pepper
- 1&1/2 cups Gruyere cheese, shredded

XXXXXXXXXXXXXXXXXXXXXXX

Instructions:

a. Turn on your oven to 375°F. Spray a 9-inch pie pan with non-stick spray.

b. Put a large non-stick pan on medium-high heat. Add olive oil and swirl it around. Throw in the mushrooms and cook for 6-8 minutes, stirring now and then, until they're brown and soft.

c. Add onions and garlic to the pan. Cook for 4-5 minutes, stirring often, until they're soft. Toss in the spinach and cook for 1-2 minutes, stirring all the time, until it wilts. Take the pan off the heat.

d. In a bowl, mix eggs, milk, half & half, Dijon mustard, thyme, salt, and pepper. Add the cheese and cooked veggies. Stir it all together.

e. Pour the mix into your pie pan. Bake for about 30 minutes until it's golden and firm.

f. Let it cool for 10-12 minutes. Sprinkle some thyme on top, cut into slices, and serve.

Special Notes:

- Try using different cheese combos for new flavors. A mix of sharp cheddar and feta works great too.
- For a crispy top, sprinkle some breadcrumbs mixed with melted butter over the pie before baking.

17. No-Sugar Fruity Oat Muffins

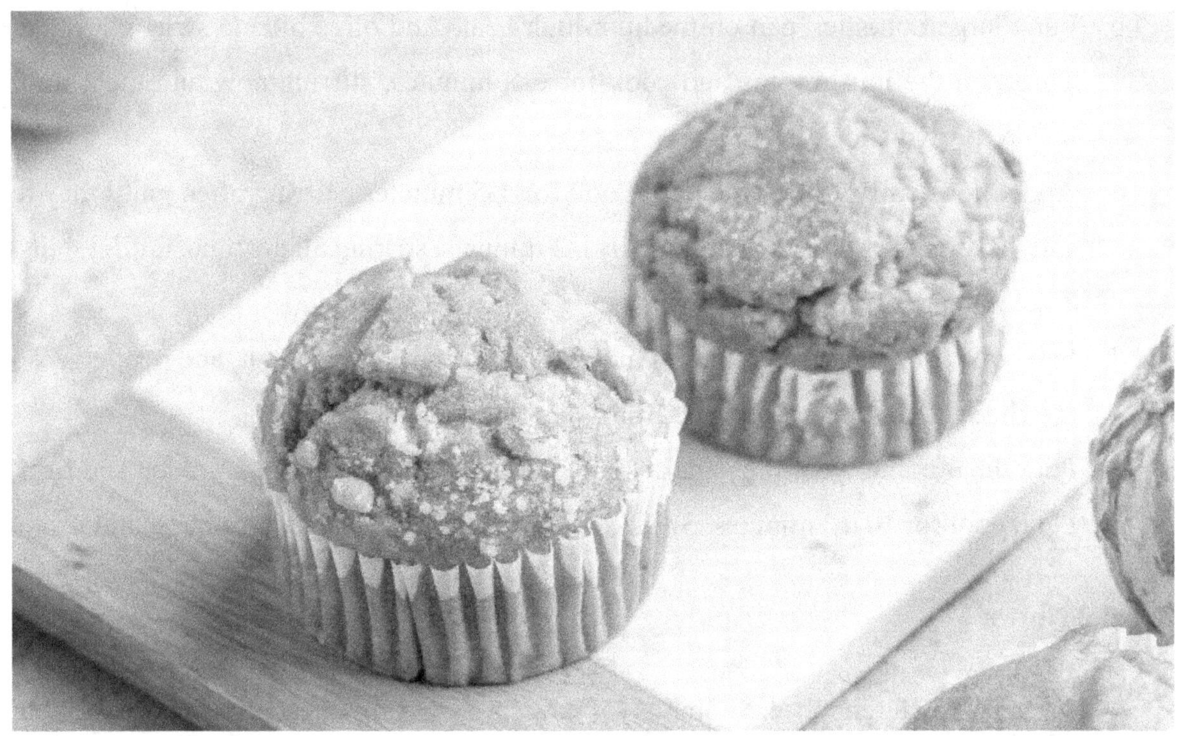

These muffins are a hit in health-conscious circles. Born in a home kitchen, they've spread like wildfire among friends and family. Packed with pears and oats, they're a tasty way to start your day. You'll love how they fill you up without weighing you down. Perfect for grab-and-go mornings!

Preparation Time: 25 minutes

Cooking Time: 30 minutes

Serving Size: 12 muffins

Ingredients:

- 4 small pears, skin-on, washed, cored, and chopped
- 1 cup rolled oats
- 1 Weetabix whole-grain cereal biscuit, crushed
- 2&1/4 cups white self-rising flour
- 2 tsp baking powder
- 1 pinch baking soda
- 1 tsp ground cinnamon
- 1/3 cup canola oil
- 2 large eggs
- 1/4 cup pure honey
- 3/4 cup low-fat milk

XXXXXXXXXXXXXXXXXXXXXXXX

Instructions:

a. Boil the pears in a pot until soft. Drain and let cool.
b. Heat your oven to 350°F.
c. Mix dry stuff in a big bowl: oats, crushed Weetabix, flour, baking soda, cinnamon, and baking powder.
d. Make a hole in the middle. Pour in milk, honey, oil, and eggs.
e. Stir the wet stuff first, then mix it all together.
f. Toss in the pear chunks and stir well.
g. Fill muffin cups to the top.
h. Bake for 25-30 minutes. They're done when they bounce back if you poke them.
i. Let them cool a bit, then pop them out and eat up!

Special Notes:

- Zap your pears in the microwave instead of boiling to save time. Just chop them up, put them in a bowl with a splash of water, cover, and microwave for 3-4 minutes.
- Try swapping half the pears for grated carrots. It adds a nice color and extra veggies to your breakfast!

18. Pumpkin Chili Cornbread Squares (Autumn Picnic Surprise)

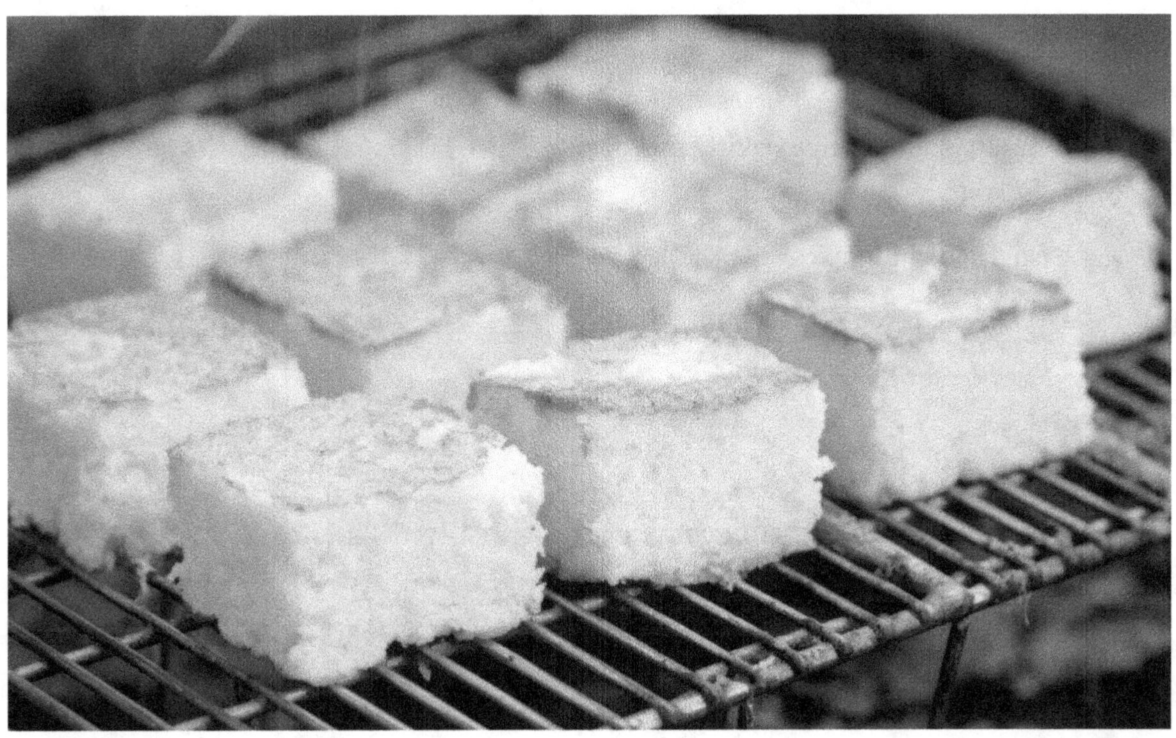

This cornbread is a family favorite for summer picnics. It's a veggie-packed twist on traditional cornbread, mixing sweet pumpkin with spicy chili flakes. The recipe comes from my grandma's old cookbook. It's easy to make and always gets people talking at potlucks.

Preparation Time: 1 hour 10 minutes

Serving size: 8 servings

Ingredients:

- 12 oz peeled butternut squash, sliced thick
- 1/2 cup olive oil
- 1&1/2 cups polenta cornmeal
- 1&1/3 cups corn flour
- 1& 1/2 tbsp maple syrup
- 1& 1/2 tsp gluten-free baking powder
- 1& 1/2 cups low-fat buttermilk
- 1 tsp dried chili flakes
- 1 cup pumpkin seeds
- 2 oz unsalted butter, melted
- 1 large egg
- Salt flakes, to taste
- Watercress sprigs for serving (optional)

xxxxxxxxxxxxxxxxxxxxxxxx

Instructions:

a. Heat oven to 400°F. Grease two big baking sheets and an 8x12-inch pan. Line them with parchment paper. Let the paper hang over the long sides of the pan.

b. Put squash on baking sheets. Add olive oil. Bake until soft, about 15 minutes.

c. Mix corn flour, polenta, baking powder, syrup, 1/2 cup pumpkin seeds, chili, and 1 tsp salt in a bowl.

d. In another bowl, mix buttermilk, egg, and melted butter. Add to the corn mix. Stir gently.

e. Put half the batter in the pan. Add a layer of squash. Top with the rest of the batter. Sprinkle remaining pumpkin seeds on top.

f. Bake for 30 minutes. Check if it's done by sticking a toothpick in the middle. If it comes out clean, it's ready.

g. Let it cool a bit. Take it out of the pan. Cut and serve warm with watercress if you like.

Special Notes:

- For extra flavor, try roasting the pumpkin seeds with a bit of smoked paprika before adding them to the batter.

- If you want a moister cornbread, add a small can of creamed corn to the batter. It'll give it a nice texture and sweetness that goes well with the chili flakes.

19. Chocolate Dream Pudding (The No-Dairy Delight)

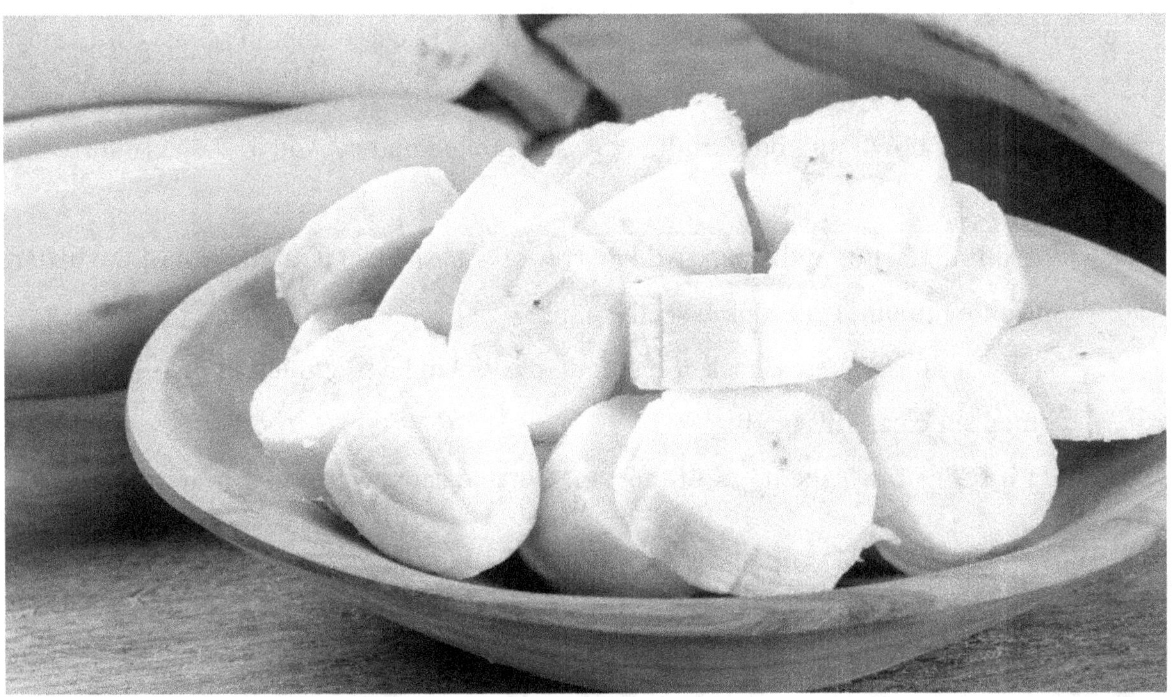

This quick and easy chocolate treat is perfect for pregnant women or anyone looking for a healthier dessert. It's a popular choice in vegan circles, using banana as the creamy base. You'll love how it satisfies your sweet tooth without any dairy.

Preparation Time: 10 minutes

Chilling Time: 45 minutes

Serving size: 1 serving

Ingredients:

- 1 ripe banana, washed
- 1 tablespoon coconut or buckwheat flour
- 1 tablespoon raw cacao powder
- 1 tablespoon maple syrup
- 1/4 teaspoon pure vanilla extract
- 2 tablespoons gluten-free coconut cream

XXXXXXXXXXXXXXXXXXXXXXXX

Instructions:

a. In a bowl, mash the banana well.
b. Add the flour, cacao powder, maple syrup, and vanilla extract to the mashed banana. Mix everything together until smooth.
c. Open a can of coconut cream. Scoop out 2 tablespoons of the thicker cream from the top.
d. Gently fold the coconut cream into the chocolate mixture. Don't mix too much - you want to keep some swirls of cream visible.
e. Put the bowl in the freezer for 30 to 45 minutes.
f. Take it out and enjoy your chilled chocolate pudding!

Special Notes:

- For extra richness, try adding a small pinch of salt to the mixture. It helps bring out the chocolate flavor even more.
- If you like some crunch, sprinkle a few cacao nibs on top just before serving. They add texture and boost the chocolatey taste without extra sugar.

20. Wonton Chicken Soup (The Slurp-tastic Broth Bowl)

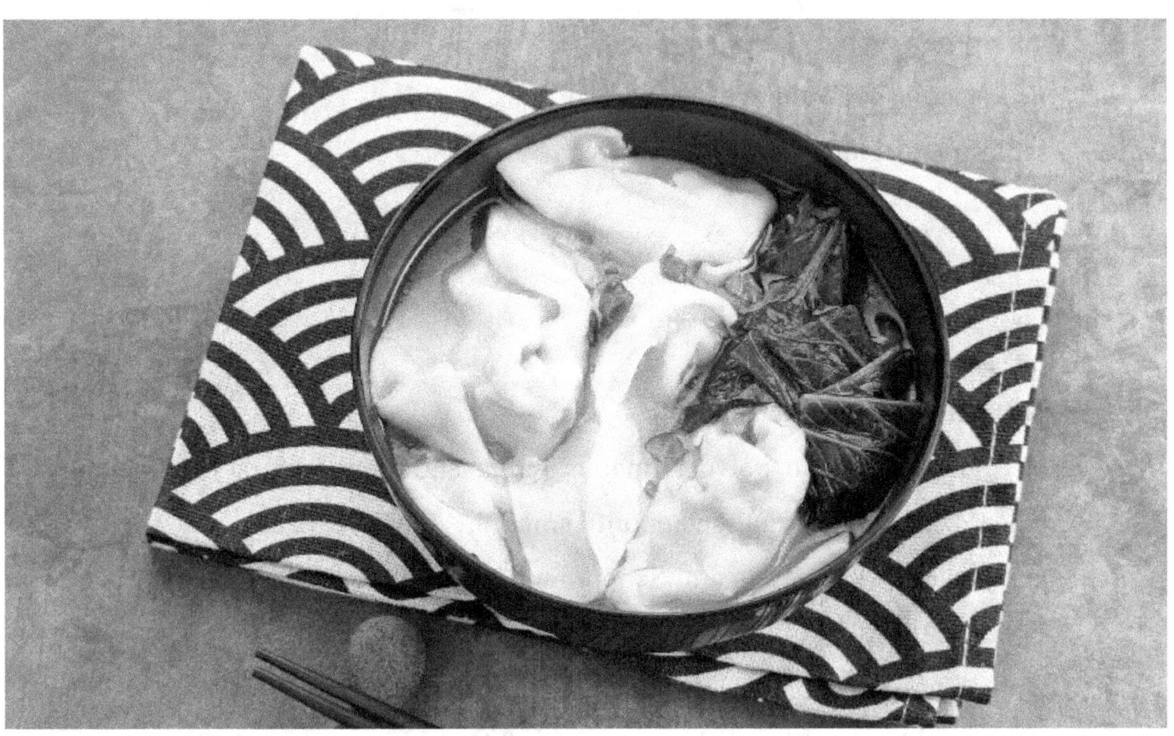

This Chinese-inspired soup is a hit in many homes. It's packed with tender chicken, veggies, and dumplings in a tasty broth. Perfect for cold nights or when you're feeling under the weather. Once you try it, you'll want to make it again and again.

Preparation Time: 30 minutes

Cooking Time: 1 hour

Serving Size: 4 servings

Ingredients:

- 2 bunches Bok choy, quartered
- 24 wonton wrappers
- 2 tablespoons vegetable oil
- 2 teaspoons sesame oil
- 1 carrot, chopped
- 1-inch piece ginger, grated
- 1/2 bunch spring onions, chopped
- 4 garlic cloves, crushed
- 4 Birdseye chilies, chopped
- 2 cups chicken stock
- 2 tablespoons Chinese rice wine
- 1/4 cup light soy sauce
- 1 whole chicken (3.5 pounds)

XXXXXXXXXXXXXXXXXXXXXXX

Instructions:

a. Heat vegetable and sesame oils in a large pot over medium heat.

b. Toss in chopped carrots, spring onions, chilies, ginger, and garlic. Cook for 2-3 minutes until soft.

c. Pour in chicken stock, rice wine, soy sauce, and 6 cups of water. Bring to a simmer.

d. Add the whole chicken, making sure it's fully covered with liquid. Simmer for about an hour until the chicken is cooked through and tender.

e. Take out the chicken and let it cool. Then shred the meat, throwing away the skin and bones.

f. Put the shredded chicken back in the pot. Add Bok choy and bring to a simmer again.

g. Drop in wonton wrappers and cook until they're soft.

h. Serve hot and enjoy your homemade wonton chicken soup!

Special Notes:

- For extra flavor, try adding a star anise pod to the broth while it simmers. Remove before serving.
- If you like it spicier, add a dollop of chili oil to each bowl when serving. It'll give your soup an extra kick!

21. Baked Apple Delight

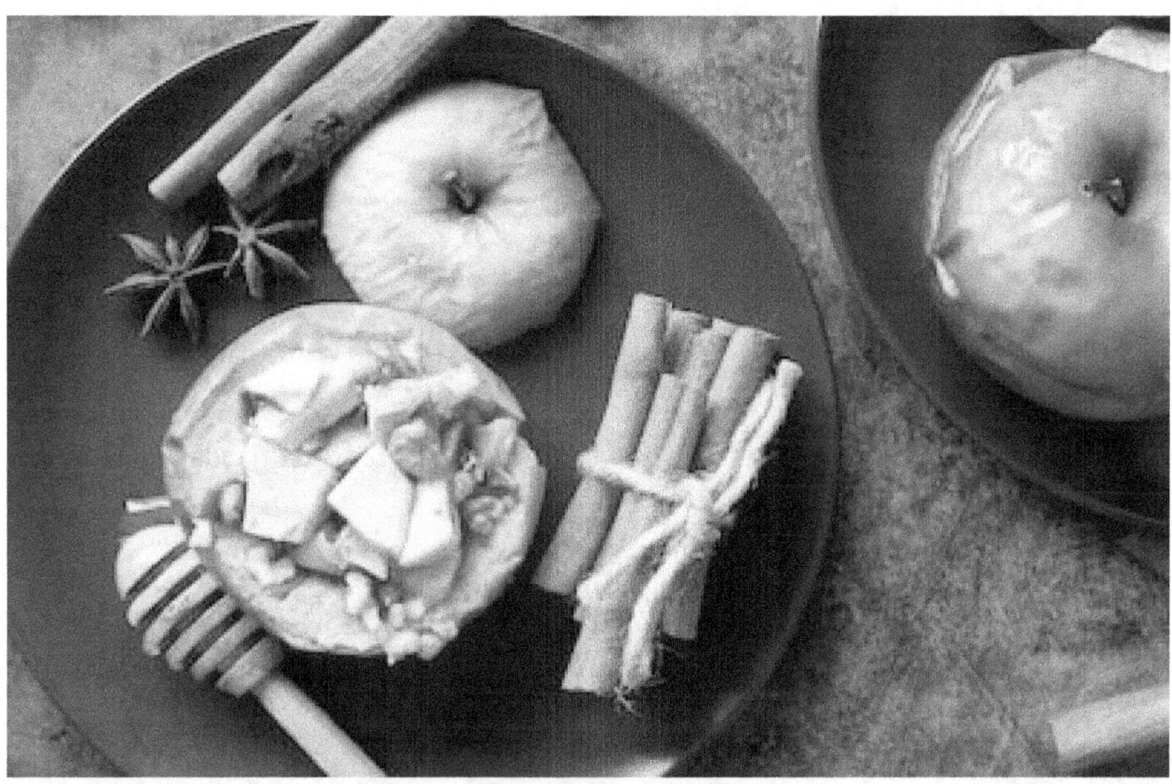

This easy-to-make treat comes from grandma's kitchen. It's a hit at family gatherings and perfect for chilly nights. The star is a juicy apple stuffed with nuts and spices. You'll love how the warm, sweet smell fills your home as it bakes.

Preparation Time: 10 minutes

Cooking Time: 4 minutes

Serving Size: 1

Ingredients:

- 1 medium red or green apple
- 1 tablespoon unsalted butter, softened
- 1/2 teaspoon ground cinnamon
- 1 tablespoon maple syrup
- 3 tablespoons chopped walnuts or pecans

xxxxxxxxxxxxxxxxxxxxxxxx

Instructions:

a. Take out the apple's core. Cut a thin slice off the bottom so it stands up. Put it in a microwave-safe bowl.
b. In a small cup, mix butter, cinnamon, syrup, and nuts.
c. Stuff the apple with the mixture. You'll have extra for later - keep it in the fridge.
d. Cover the apple with plastic wrap. Microwave on high for 3-4 minutes until soft.
e. Let it cool a bit, then dig in!

Special Notes:

- For a twist, add a pinch of cardamom to the filling. It gives a subtle, exotic flavor that pairs well with the apple.
- If you like a crispy top, finish the apple under the broiler for 1-2 minutes. Watch it closely to avoid burning!

22. Beefy Veggie Soup - The Winter Warmer

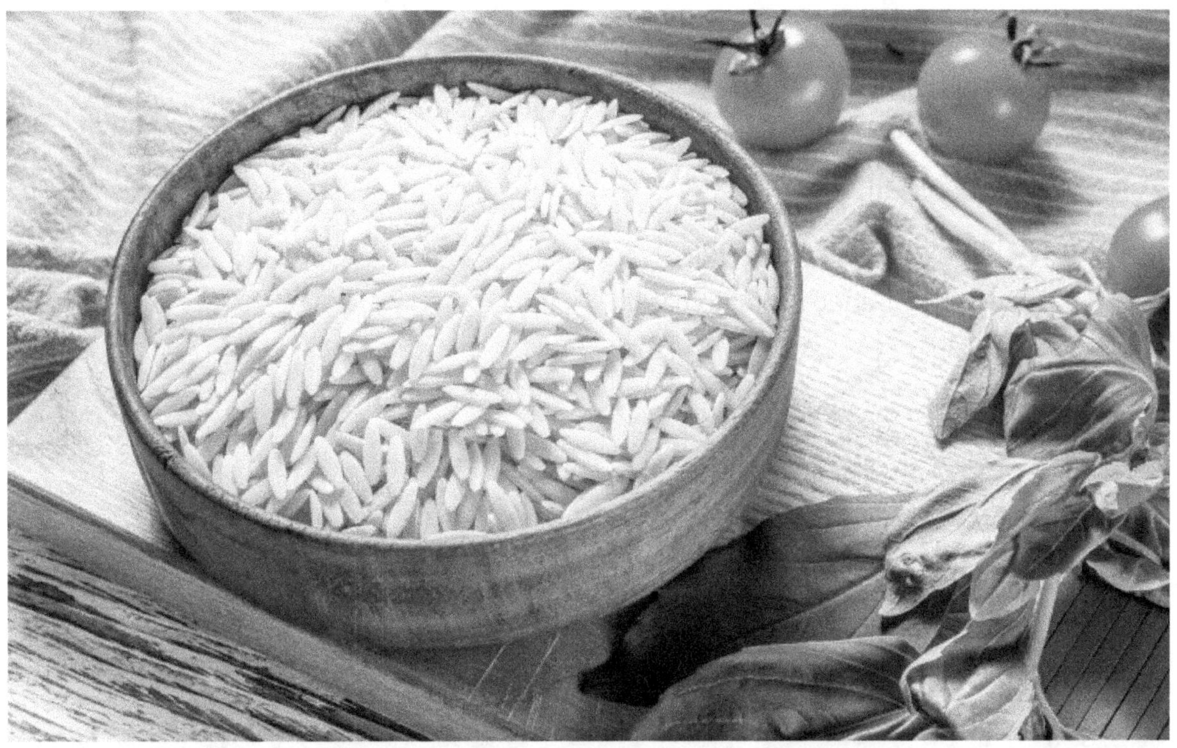

This Italian soup is a hit in cold weather. It's packed with beef, veggies, and pasta. People love it because it's filling and tasty. You'll find it in many homes and restaurants in Italy. It's perfect for lunch or dinner when you want something hot and hearty.

Preparation Time: 3 hours 15 minutes

Serving size: 6 servings

Ingredients:

- 1 pound beef, trimmed and chopped into 3/4-inch pieces
- 2 garlic cloves, finely chopped
- 2 carrots, finely chopped
- 2 celery stalks, finely chopped
- 2 tablespoons olive oil
- 1 medium onion, finely chopped
- 1/3 cup no-salt-added tomato paste
- 1/2 cup red wine
- 1 can (14 oz) chopped tomatoes
- 4 cups beef stock
- 5 oz orzo pasta
- 5 oz baby spinach leaves

To serve:

- Parmesan cheese
- Pesto

XXXXXXXXXXXXXXXXXXXXXXX

Instructions:

a. Pour oil in a big pot. Heat it up on medium-high.

b. Put some salt and pepper on the beef. Cook it in small batches. Each batch should take about 3-4 minutes. Stir it now and then until it turns brown. Take the beef out and set it aside.

c. Throw in the carrots, garlic, onion, and celery. Cook and stir for 4-5 minutes until they get soft.

d. Put the beef back in. Add tomato paste and cook for a minute while stirring.

e. Pour in the stock, tomatoes, and wine. Add salt and pepper if you want. Let it start to bubble, then turn the heat down low. Put a lid on, but not all the way.

f. Let it cook for about 2 hours. The beef should get really soft.

g. Add the orzo pasta. Cook for about 10 minutes until it's not too hard, not too soft.

h. Mix in the spinach and stir until it shrinks down.

i. Scoop the soup into bowls. Top with some Parmesan and pesto if you like.

j. Eat up!

Special Notes:

- Try adding a splash of balsamic vinegar at the end. It gives a nice tangy kick.
- If you like it spicy, throw in a pinch of red pepper flakes with the veggies. It'll warm you up even more!

23. Spicy Chicken Rice Bowl

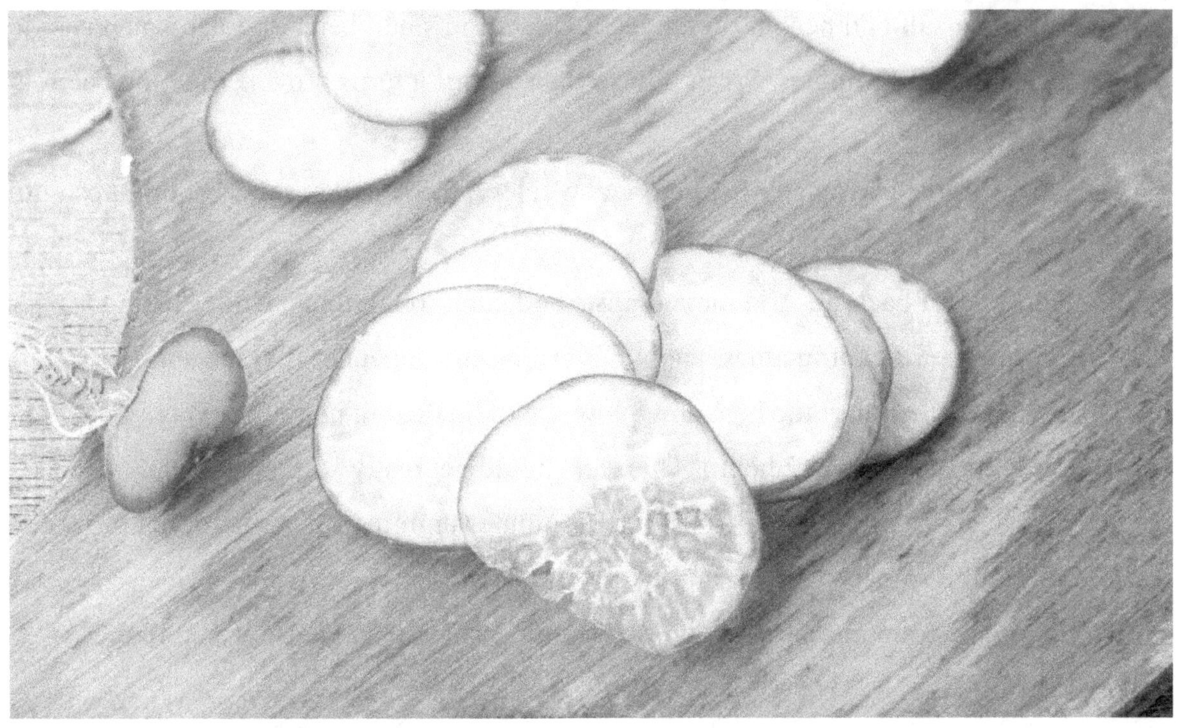

This Korean-inspired dish is a hit in many homes. It's a tasty mix of spicy chicken, rice, and fresh toppings. The gochujang (Korean chili paste) gives it a kick, while the pears add a sweet crunch. It's easy to make and perfect for a quick dinner.

Preparation Time: 35 minutes

Serving size: 4 servings

Ingredients:

- 8 skinless chicken thigh fillets
- 1/4 cup Korean fermented chili paste (gochujang)
- 2 tablespoons olive oil
- 1 pound microwave brown or black rice
- 1/2 teaspoon sesame oil
- 1 teaspoon low-sodium soy sauce
- 1/2 crushed garlic clove
- 2 pears, cut into matchsticks
- 3 radishes, thinly sliced
- 2/3 cup kimchi
- 1 cup loosely packed baby spinach
- 1 cup loosely packed Thai basil leaves
- 4 large eggs, fried (for serving)
- Shiso herb leaves, to taste
- White and black toasted sesame seeds (for serving)

xxxxxxxxxxxxxxxxxxxxxxxx

Instructions:

a. Mix the chicken with olive oil and chili paste in a bowl.

b. Heat a grill pan on high. Cook the chicken for 2-3 minutes on one side, then 4-5 minutes on the other until done. Set aside and cover to keep warm.

c. Cook the rice as per package instructions. Put it in a bowl and mix in the sesame oil, soy sauce, and garlic.

d. Cut the cooked chicken into thin slices.

e. Divide the rice among four bowls. Top each with chicken, pears, radishes, kimchi, shiso, basil, and spinach.

f. Add a fried egg to each bowl. Sprinkle with sesame seeds and serve.

Special Notes:

- For extra flavor, marinate the chicken in the chili paste mix for 30 minutes before cooking.
- Try swapping the pears for green apples for a tart twist. It pairs well with the spicy chicken and adds a nice crunch.

24. Chicken Veggie Tortilla Melt

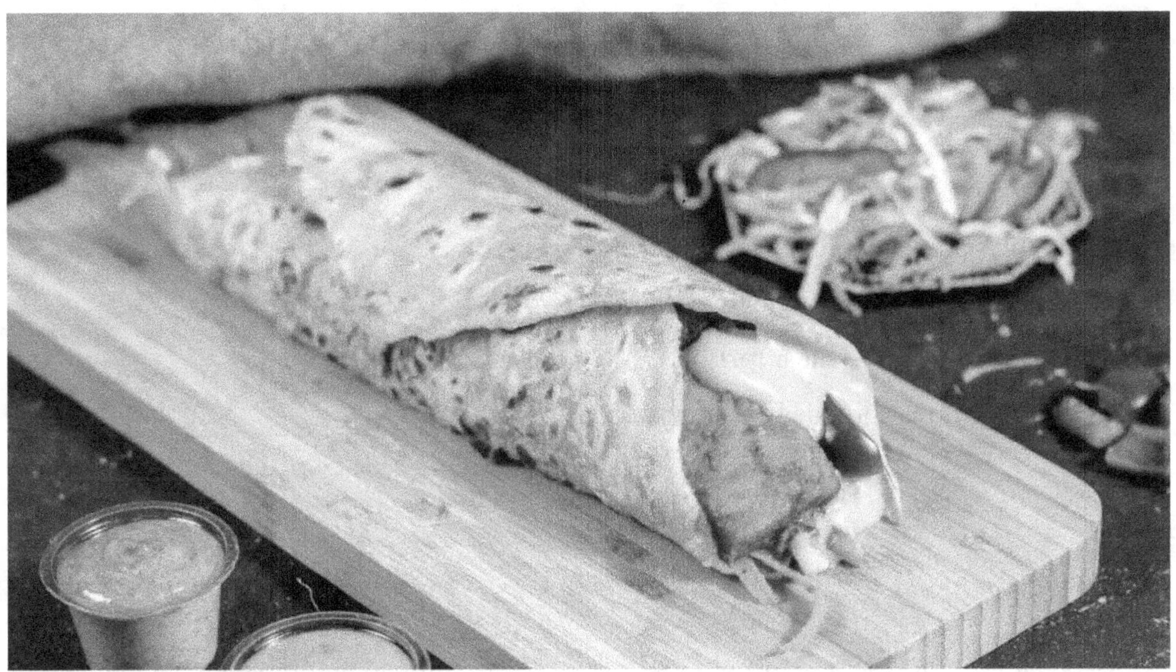

This quick and easy Mexican-inspired dish is a hit in many American homes. It's a great way to use up leftover chicken or turkey. The mix of veggies and melted cheese in a crispy tortilla makes it a tasty lunch or light dinner. You'll love how fast it comes together!

Preparation Time: 25 minutes

Serving size: 1 serving

Ingredients:

- 2 teaspoons canola oil
- 1/4 cup chopped onion
- 1/4 cup diced red bell pepper
- 1/4 cup diced zucchini
- 2 oz shredded cooked chicken
- 2 tablespoons whole kernel corn (frozen and rinsed, or fresh)
- 1 tablespoon fresh chopped cilantro (optional)
- 1 (8-inch) whole-wheat tortilla
- 3 tablespoons shredded pepper jack cheese

xxxxxxxxxxxxxxxxxxxxxxxx

Instructions:

a. Heat oil in a skillet over medium heat. Toss in onions, bell peppers, and zucchini. Cook for 3-4 minutes, stirring often, until veggies soften.

b. Add chicken and corn. Cook for about a minute until everything's hot. If using cilantro, mix it in now. Scoop the veggie mix into a small bowl. Clean and dry the skillet.

c. Lay the tortilla on a cutting board. Sprinkle 1 tablespoon of cheese on half the tortilla, leaving a 1/2 inch edge. Top with the veggie mix and the rest of the cheese. Fold the tortilla in half.

d. Heat the clean skillet over medium heat. Add the folded tortilla and cook for 1-2 minutes on each side. The cheese should melt and the tortilla should turn brown.

e. Cut into three wedges and serve hot.

Special Notes:

- For extra crunch, try adding a handful of crushed tortilla chips to the veggie mix before folding the quesadilla.
- If you like it spicy, mix a dash of hot sauce or a pinch of chili flakes into the veggie mixture for a fiery kick.

25. Harvest Turkey Chili (The Pumpkin Surprise)

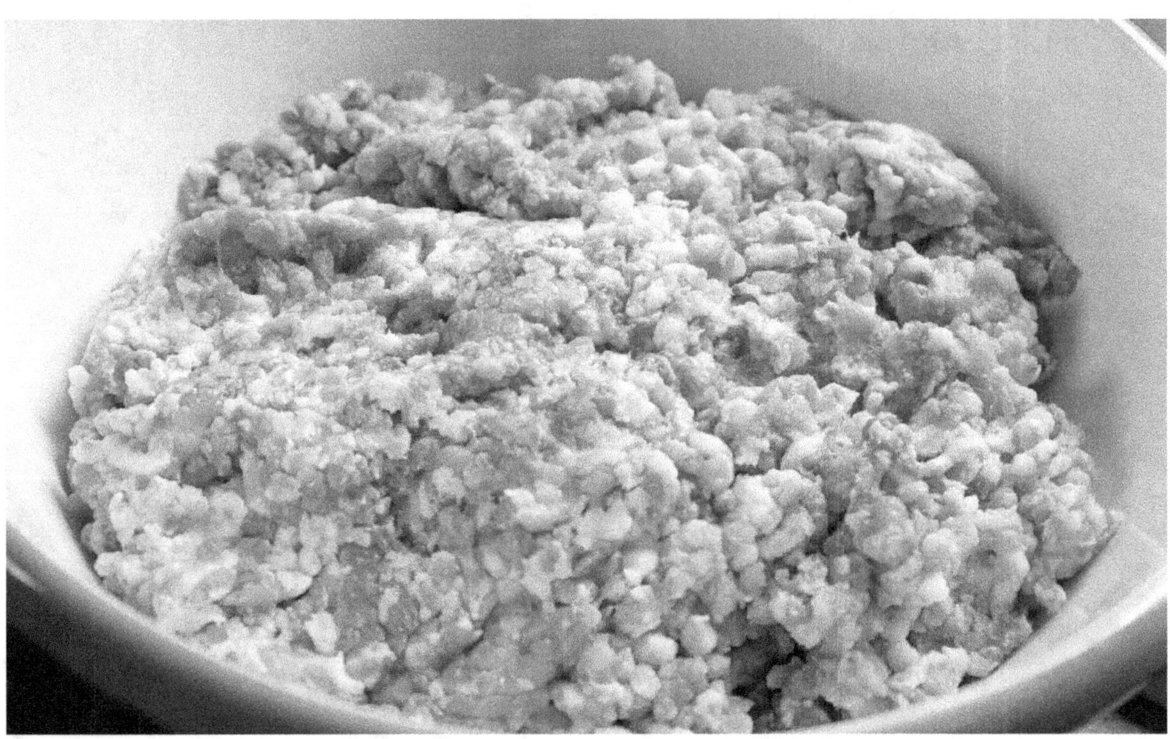

This hearty chili comes from the American Southwest. It's a fall favorite that blends turkey and pumpkin for a unique twist. The mix of spices gives it a warm kick, perfect for chilly evenings. You'll love how the pumpkin adds thickness without overpowering the classic chili taste.

Preparation Time: 40 minutes

Serving size: 4 servings

Ingredients:

- 2 cups packed chopped kale leaves
- 4 tablespoons light sour cream
- 1 tablespoon olive oil
- 1 medium yellow onion, chopped
- 1 small green bell pepper, chopped
- 3 garlic cloves, minced
- 1 pound ground turkey
- 1 (14.5 oz) can fire-roasted diced tomatoes with juices
- 1 (15 oz) can black beans, no salt added, rinsed
- 1 (15 oz) can unseasoned pumpkin puree
- 1 1/2 cups filtered water
- 1 tablespoon chili powder
- 1 1/2 teaspoons ground cumin
- 1 teaspoon smoked paprika
- 1/4 teaspoon ground pepper
- 1/8 teaspoon kosher salt
- Fresh chopped cilantro for garnish (optional)

XXXXXXXXXXXXXXXXXXXXXXXX

Instructions:

a. Get a large pot hot over medium-high heat. Pour in the oil, then toss in the onion, bell pepper, and garlic. Cook for about 5 minutes, stirring often, until they're just starting to soften.

b. Add the ground turkey. Break it up with a spoon and cook until it's no longer pink, about 5 minutes.

c. Dump in the tomatoes, beans, pumpkin, water, and all the spices.

d. Give it a good stir and bring it to a boil.

e. Turn the heat down low, put a lid on it, and let it simmer for about 20 minutes. Stir it now and then.

f. In the last 5 minutes, throw in the kale and stir it in.

g. Serve it up in bowls. Top each with a spoonful of sour cream and some cilantro if you like.

Special Notes:

- For extra flavor, try roasting the pumpkin seeds and using them as a crunchy topping.
- If you like it spicier, add a diced jalapeño with the bell pepper or stir in some hot sauce at the end.

26. Veggie-Packed Lentil Stew (The Cozy Bowl)

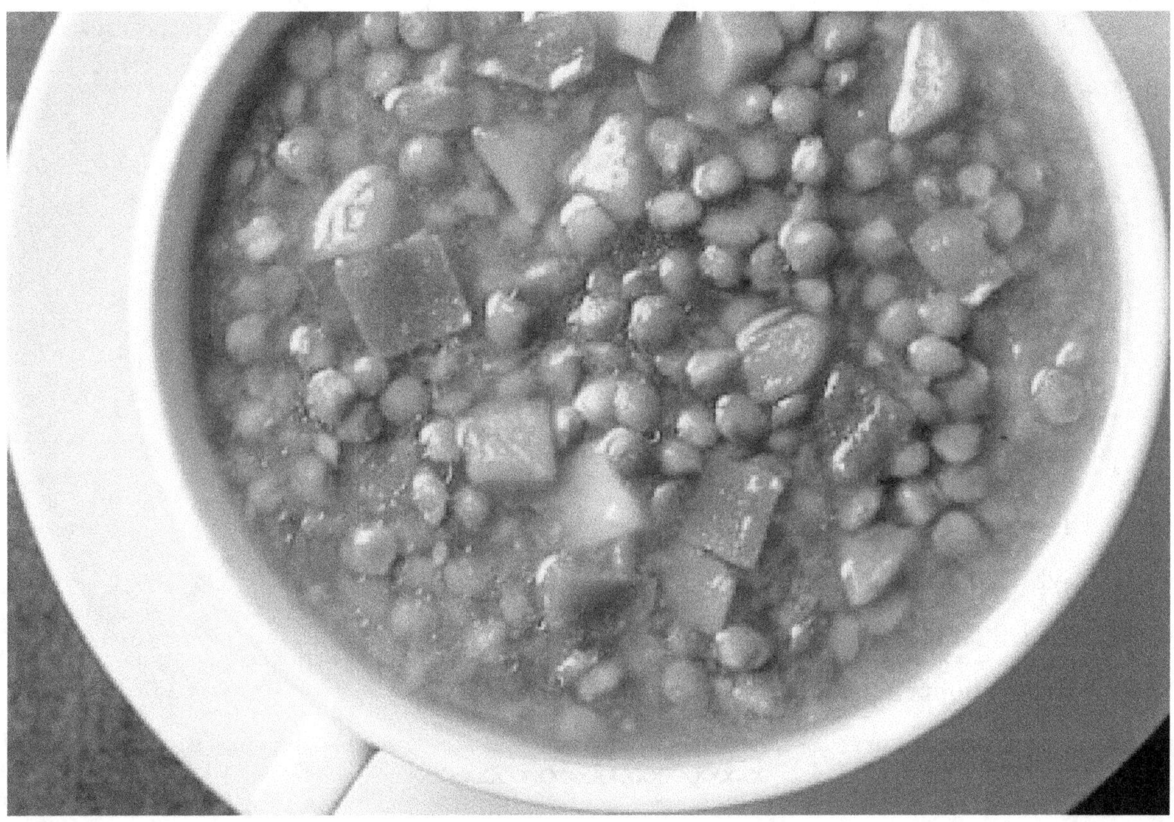

This tasty lentil stew comes from Italy. It's a hit with folks who like hearty meals. The main stars are lentils, veggies, and herbs. You'll love how it warms you up and fills you up. It's perfect for cold days or when you need a quick, healthy meal.

Preparation Time: 15 minutes

Cooking Time: 45 minutes

Serving Size: 6 servings

Ingredients:

- 3 cups mixed chopped celery, onion, and carrot (frozen or fresh)
- 3 cups roughly chopped and packed Lacinato kale
- 4 garlic cloves, chopped
- 4 cups low-sodium chicken or vegetable broth
- 1 can (15 oz) no-salt-added diced tomatoes with juice
- 2 tablespoons olive oil
- 2 teaspoons finely chopped fresh thyme
- 1/2 teaspoon kosher salt
- 1/2 teaspoon ground pepper
- 1/2 teaspoon crushed red pepper
- 1/2 cup grated Parmesan cheese
- 1&1/2 cups brown or green lentils
- 1&1/2 tablespoons red wine vinegar
- Fresh chopped parsley for garnish (optional)

XXXXXXXXXXXXXXXXXXXXXXX

Instructions:

a. Get a big pot. Put it on the stove. Turn the heat to medium.

b. Pour in the olive oil. Add the veggie mix. Cook for 6-9 minutes. Stir now and then. The veggies should get soft.

c. Toss in the garlic. Cook for 30 seconds. Keep stirring. It should smell good.

d. Now add the broth, tomatoes, lentils, thyme, salt, pepper, and red pepper. Stir it all up.

e. Turn the heat up. Wait for it to boil. Then turn the heat down to medium-low.

f. Put a lid on the pot. Let it cook for 15-25 minutes. Stir sometimes. The lentils should be almost soft. Add water if you want the soup thinner.

g. Put in the kale. Stir well. Cover again. Cook for 5-10 minutes until the kale is soft.

h. Add the vinegar. Stir it in.

i. Serve the soup in bowls. Put some cheese on top. Add parsley if you want.

Special Notes:

- Try soaking the lentils for a few hours before cooking. This makes them cook faster and can help with digestion.

- For a smoky flavor, add a teaspoon of smoked paprika when you put in the broth. It gives the stew a nice twist without changing the recipe too much.

27. Zesty Pork Guac Stack (The Avocado Porker's Dream)

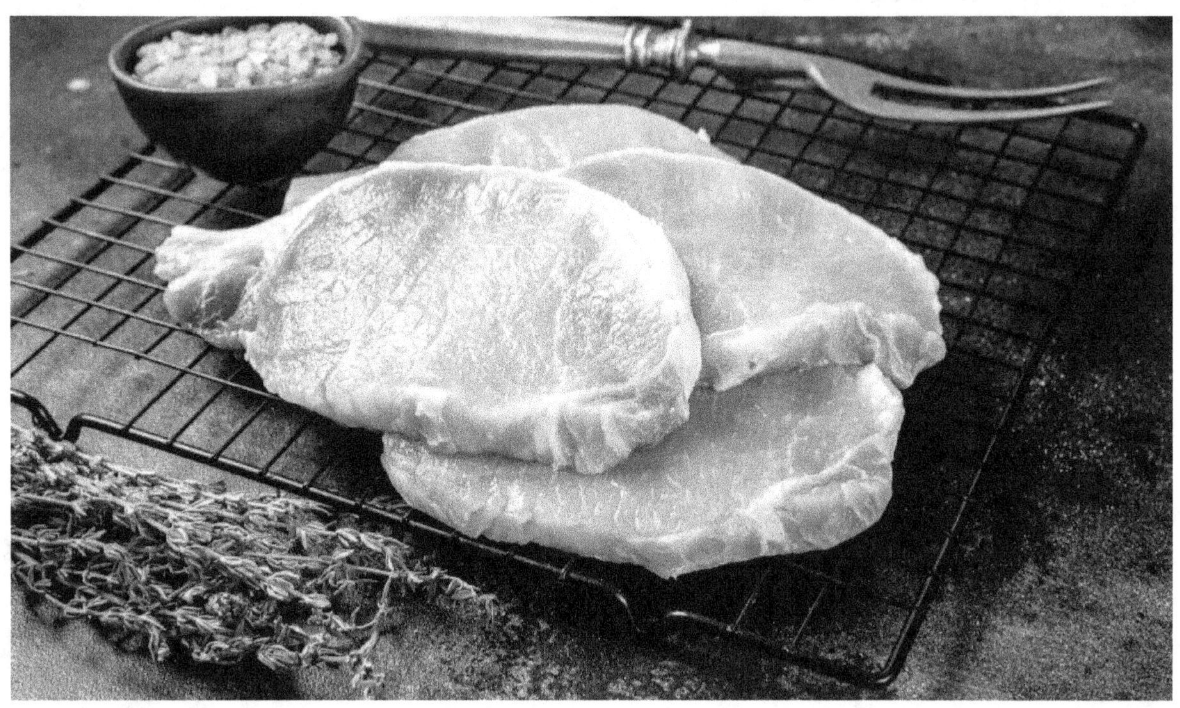

This Mexican-inspired dish is a hit in Texas. It's a quick meal that combines juicy pork with creamy guacamole. The marinade gives the pork a spicy kick, while the fresh guacamole cools things down. It's perfect for busy weeknights or casual get-togethers with friends.

Preparation Time: 25 minutes

Serving size: 4 servings

Ingredients:

- 4 pork cutlets, trimmed
- 1/2 cup peri-peri marinade
- 1 baby cos lettuce, leaves separated
- 1 tablespoon olive oil
- 2 limes, halved (for serving)

For the guacamole:

- 1 avocado, flesh only
- 1 tablespoon lime juice (about 1/2 lime)
- 1/4 cup roughly chopped coriander leaves

xxxxxxxxxxxxxxxxxxxxxxxx

Instructions:

a. Pound the pork cutlets to about 3/4 inch thick using a meat mallet.
b. Coat the pork with the peri-peri marinade and let it sit for 5-7 minutes.
c. Make the guacamole: Mash the avocado in a bowl. Mix in the lime juice and coriander. Add salt and pepper to taste.
d. Toss lettuce with 1/2 tablespoon olive oil in a separate dish. Season the dish with salt and pepper.
e. Heat the remaining olive oil in a large non-stick pan over medium-high heat.
f. Cook the pork for 4-5 minutes on each side until medium done.
g. Turn off the heat, cover the pan, and let the pork rest for 4-7 minutes.
h. Serve the pork with the guacamole, lettuce leaves, and lime halves on the side.

- For extra tang, grate some lime zest into the guacamole.
- Try using different lettuce varieties like butter lettuce or romaine for a change in texture and flavor.

28. Lemon Squares

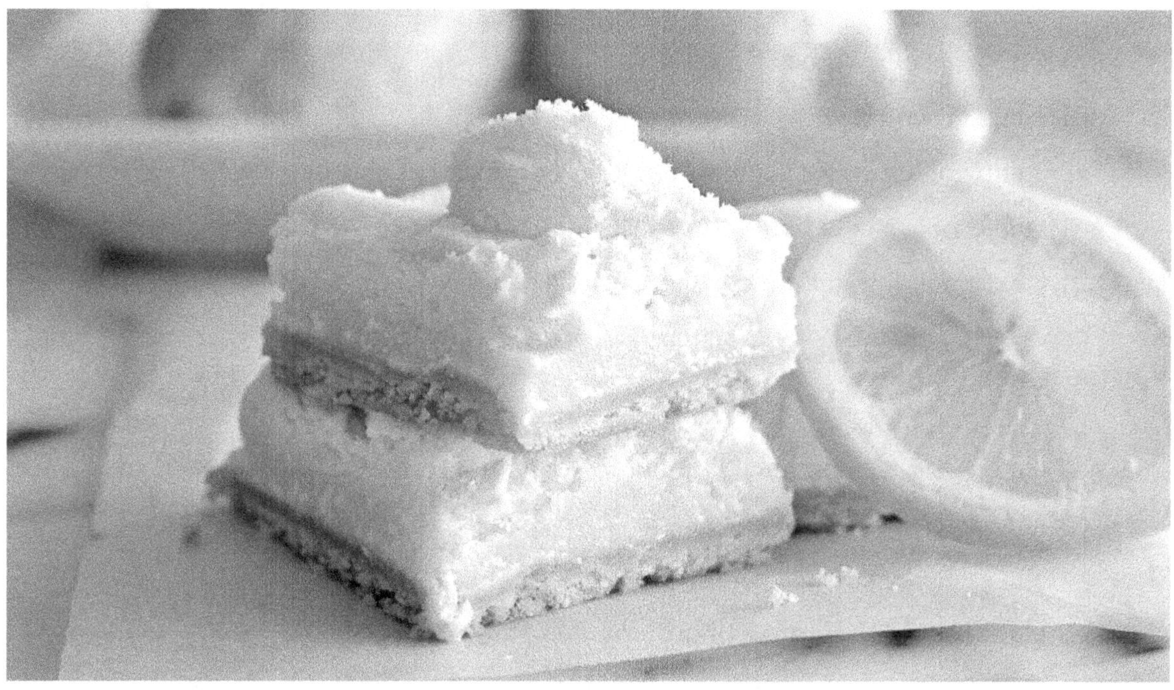

These little lemon squares are a hit at parties. They're from the UK and people love them. The main ingredients are lemons, eggs, and flour. You'll enjoy the mix of sweet and tangy flavors. They're easy to make and great for sharing.

Preparation Time: 1 hour 10 minutes

Serving size: 16 squares

Ingredients:

For the base:

- 1&1/2 cups all-purpose flour
- 1/3 cup ground rice
- 2/3 cup golden caster sugar
- 10 tablespoons cold butter, diced
- 1 tablespoon low-fat milk

For the lemon topping:

- 3 lemons, zested and juiced (about 3/4 cup juice)
- 3 large eggs
- 1 cup caster sugar
- 3 tablespoons all-purpose flour

For dusting:

- Powdered sugar, as needed

XXXXXXXXXXXXXXXXXXXXXXXX

Instructions:

a. Heat your oven to 400°F. Put parchment paper in a 9-inch square baking pan.

b. Mix flour, ground rice, and sugar in a bowl. Add butter and rub it in until it looks like breadcrumbs.

c. Stir in the milk. Press the mix into the pan evenly.

d. Bake for 15-20 minutes until it's light brown. Take it out and turn the oven down to 350°F.

e. In another bowl, mix eggs and lemon juice. Strain this into a bowl with the lemon zest, sugar, and flour. Whisk it all together.

f. Pour this mix over the baked base. Bake again for 10-15 minutes until the top is set.

g. Let it cool in the pan. Sprinkle powdered sugar on top, then cut into squares.

Special Notes:

- For extra zing, grate a bit of fresh ginger into the lemon topping mixture.
- Try using Meyer lemons if you can find them. They're sweeter and give a unique flavor to the bars.

29. Stir-Fried Pork Noodle Bowl

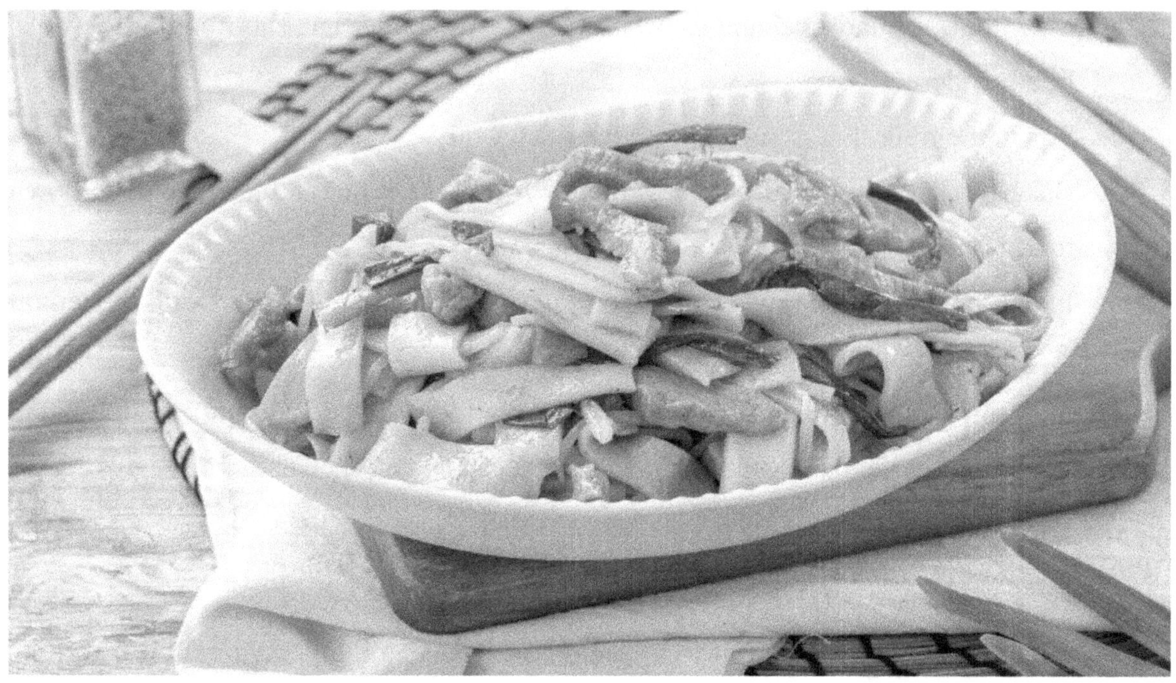

This tasty dish mixes juicy pork with tangy pickled cucumbers. It's a popular meal in many Asian homes. The mix of textures - from soft noodles to crisp veggies - makes it fun to eat. You'll love how the flavors blend together. It's quick to make and perfect for busy weeknights.

Preparation Time: 35 minutes

Serving size: 4 servings

Ingredients:

- 1 cucumber (Lebanese if you can find it)
- 1/2 teaspoon sugar
- 1 red chili, seeds removed and chopped
- 4 tablespoons rice vinegar
- 2 tablespoons soy sauce
- 2 tablespoons oyster sauce
- 1 tablespoon sweet chili sauce
- 1 tablespoon cornstarch
- 2 cups water
- 2 teaspoons fresh grated ginger
- 3 spring onions, thinly sliced
- 1 pound ground pork, lean
- 5 ounces snow peas, cut diagonally
- 1/3 cup coriander leaves
- 5 ounces rice noodles

XXXXXXXXXXXXXXXXXXXXXXXX

Instructions:

a. Peel the cucumber into long, thin strips. Throw away the seedy center.

b. Mix chili, 2 tablespoons vinegar, and sugar in a bowl. Stir until sugar dissolves. Add cucumber strips and set aside.

c. In another bowl, mix soy sauce, oyster sauce, sweet chili sauce, and 2 cups water. In a small bowl, mix cornstarch with 2 tablespoons vinegar.

d. Heat oil in a wok over medium-high heat. Cook spring onions and ginger for 30 seconds until fragrant.

e. Add pork to the wok. Cook and stir for 4-5 minutes until browned.

f. Pour in the sauce mix. Cook for 1-2 minutes. Add snow peas and stir-fry for 1-2 minutes until just tender.

g. Mix in coriander.

h. Cook rice noodles following package instructions.

i. Put noodles in four bowls. Top with pork mix and pickled cucumbers.

Special Notes:

- Try adding a tablespoon of peanut butter to the sauce for extra richness and nutty flavor.
- For a veggie boost, toss in a handful of bean sprouts just before serving. They'll add a nice crunch!

30. No-Sugar Fudge Squares

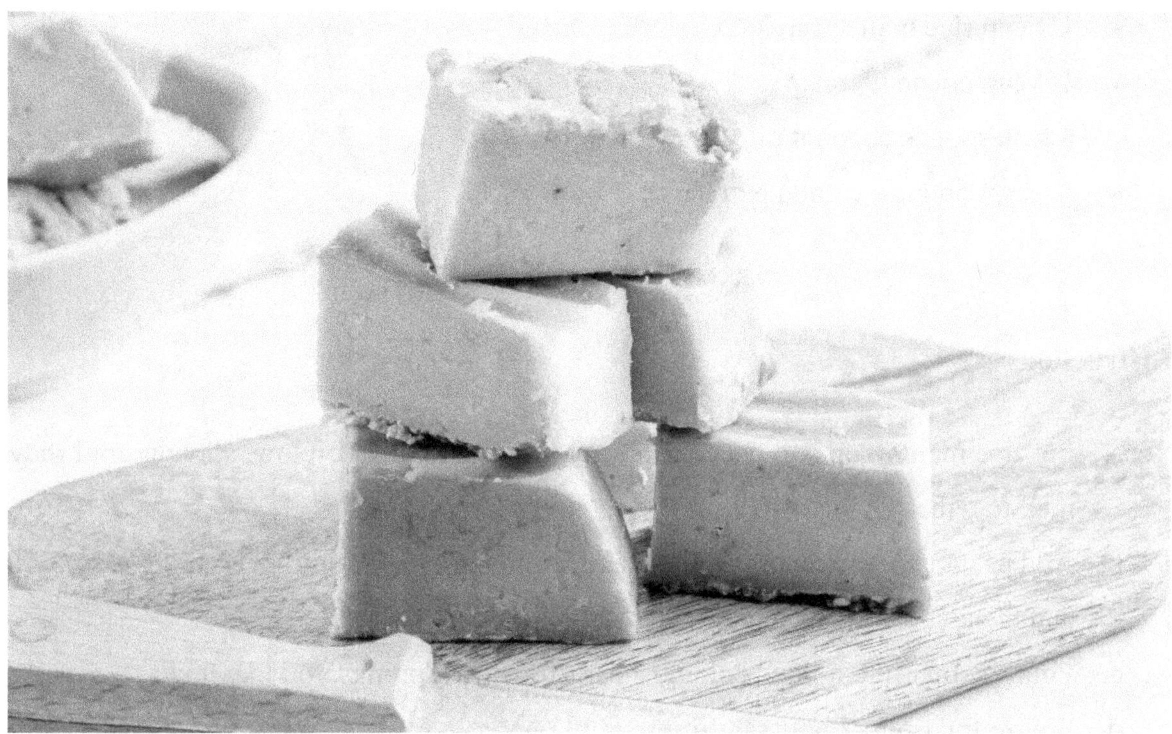

This sugar-free fudge is a hit at parties and potlucks. Made with peanut butter and coconut cream, it's a rich treat without the guilt. People love its smooth texture and natural sweetness. It's perfect for anyone watching their sugar intake but still craving something decadent.

Preparation Time: 2 hours 20 minutes

Serving size: 24 bite-sized pieces

Ingredients:

- 16 oz (1 jar) smooth peanut butter
- 1/2 cup rice malt syrup
- 1/4 cup coconut cream
- 3 tablespoons coconut oil
- 1 teaspoon pure vanilla extract

XXXXXXXXXXXXXXXXXXXXXXX

Instructions:

a. Put rice malt syrup and coconut oil in a small pot. Heat on low, stirring until they melt together.
b. Add peanut butter, coconut cream, and vanilla. Mix well until everything is smooth and blended.
c. Pour the mix into a lined baking sheet. Add any toppings you like now.
d. Freeze for 1.5 to 2 hours until set.
e. Cut into small squares and enjoy!

Special Notes:

- For extra crunch, sprinkle some chopped peanuts or shredded coconut on top before freezing.
- Try swirling in a tablespoon of unsweetened cocoa powder for a chocolate twist. It adds flavor without sugar!

Conclusion

Now you have a whole range of tasty, healthy recipes to try during your pregnancy! This book has shown you how to mix different ingredients to make dishes that are both good for you and full of flavor.

You've learned how to add high-nutrient meals to your everyday cooking. You can make simple but delicious salads like cucumber salad and chicken cobb salad. These aren't just tasty - they're packed with good things for you and your baby.

For colder days, you now know how to cook warm, comforting soups and stews. These aren't just cozy - they're full of nutrients that your growing baby needs.

You've also discovered how to prepare seafood dishes that are safe and healthy for pregnancy. Fish like salmon and catfish are great to eat all year round and offer important nutrients.

The book has taught you how to use potatoes and pasta in nutritious ways. These filling ingredients can be part of many comforting, healthy meals.

And let's not forget about desserts! You can now make treats like lemon bars and chocolate mousse that are both yummy and suitable for pregnancy. These are perfect for sharing with friends and family.

Remember, eating well during pregnancy doesn't have to be boring or difficult. With these recipes, you can enjoy delicious meals that are good for both you and your baby. Happy cooking, and enjoy this special time!

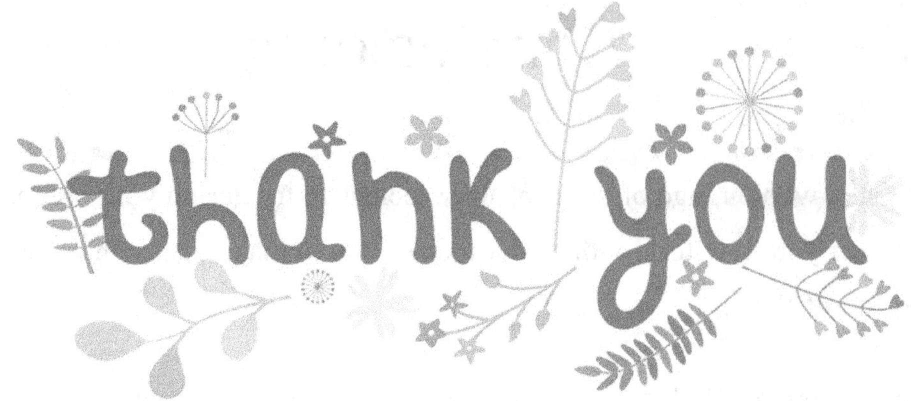

Dear Reader,

I want to express my sincere gratitude for downloading and dedicating your time to reading my book. It means the world to me that you chose to invest your valuable time in exploring the content I have shared. I truly hope that you found the information beneficial and that you had an enjoyable reading experience.

As an author, my primary goal is to impart my knowledge and insights to others. I recognize that there is an overwhelming number of e-books available, and I am deeply honored that you decided to give mine a chance. Your decision to read my work reflects your commitment to personal growth and learning, and I am thrilled to have played a role in your journey.

If you could spare a moment to provide an honest review or feedback about my book, I would be incredibly grateful. Your opinions and suggestions are invaluable to my development as a writer. They help me understand what resonates with readers and inspire me to create even more valuable content in the future. Who knows, your feedback might even spark the idea for my next book!

Once again, thank you for your support and dedication. It means more to me than words can express.

Martha Stanford